True or false?

Back pain is just a fa[c]... in medication to get relief.

False. Back pain can [be] ...[reli]eved by following proven, integrative treatment programs, most of which do not require the use of pain medications or invasive procedures.

The only way to diagnose back problems is through X-rays, MRIs, and other expensive tests.

False. X-rays and other imaging tests are usually unnecessary and can produce false diagnoses. A thorough physical exam, combined with patient input, is usually all it takes to diagnose a back problem.

When you have a bad back, you should avoid physical activity.

False. The right kind of exercise program is key to your recovery from back pain. Other therapies, including pain medication, are supplemental.

Most back pain sufferers do not receive the treatment they need because it is never offered to them.

True. All too often a complaint about back pain is answered with a prescription for pain killers and a warning to "be careful." To get the relief you need, you must educate yourself and take the initiative in developing your treatment and prevention program.

TAKE CONTROL OF YOUR LIFE AND
FIND LASTING RELIEF WITH . . .

WHAT YOUR DOCTOR MAY NOT TELL YOU ABOUT™ BACK PAIN

WHAT YOUR DOCTOR MAY *NOT* TELL YOU ABOUT™

BACK PAIN

The 6-Step Program for Lasting Relief

DEBRA K. WEINER, M.D.

with

DEBORAH MITCHELL

Paula Breuer, consulting editor

A Lynn Sonberg Book

WARNER
WELLNESS

NEW YORK   BOSTON

PUBLISHER'S NOTE: The information herein is not intended to replace the services of trained health professionals or be a substitute for medical advice. You are advised to consult with your health care professional with regard to matters relating to your health, and in particular regarding matters that may require diagnosis or medical attention.

Warner Wellness
Hachette Book Group USA
237 Park Avenue
New York, NY 10169
Visit our Web site at www.HachetteBookGroupUSA.com.

Warner Wellness is an imprint of Warner Books.

Printed in the United States of America

First Edition: April 2007
10 9 8 7 6 5 4 3 2 1

Warner Wellness is a trademark of Time Warner Inc. or an affiliated company. Used under license by Hachette Book Group USA, which is not affiliated with Time Warner Inc.

Library of Congress Cataloging-in-Publication Data
Weiner, Debra K.
    What your doctor may not tell you about back pain : the 6-step program for lasting relief / Debra K. Weiner and Deborah Mitchell. — 1st ed.
        p. cm.
    Includes index.
    ISBN-13: 978-0-446-69495-7
    ISBN-10: 0-446-69495-9
    1. Backache—Treatment—Popular works. 2. Back—Care and hygiene—Popular works. I. Mitchell, Deborah R.   II. Title.
    RD771.B217W46   2007
    617.5'64—dc22
                                                                    2006027615

Book design by Charles A. Sutherland

It is with much love and appreciation that I dedicate this book to my husband, Neal Samuels, for his unconditional support.

Acknowledgments

⸎

This book resulted from the guidance, tutelage, and support of a wide variety of individuals whose paths I have had the good fortune to cross over many years—department chairmen, teachers, patients, research study participants, family, and friends. Without them, its conceptualization and creation would not have been possible. I want to especially acknowledge Dr. Neil Resnick, my division chief at the University of Pittsburgh School of Medicine ("Pitt"); Dr. Mark Zeidel, former chairman of the Department of Medicine; and Dr. Eric Rodriguez who recruited me to come to Pitt in 1998. Their combined steadfast support and guidance has been an invaluable component of my career development.

Several colleagues provided critical feedback during the book's development, and to them I am very grateful. Paula Breuer, consulting editor and the physical therapist at our inter-disciplinary pain clinic, very carefully reviewed and revised the first four chapters. Her expertise on chronic pain is unique among the many physical therapists with whom I have worked, and she has been a motivating force behind my clinical, teaching, and research interests in chronic low back pain. Raymond Hanlon, the psychologist at our clinic, reviewed the chapter "Minding Your Back" and provided many useful suggestions. Dr. Natalia Morone's expertise in mindfulness meditation was key in ensuring the relevance and accuracy of this section in chapter 5. I also need to acknowledge colleagues who have played a pivotal role in my career and without whom this book may never have been conceived. Thomas Rudy, psychologist and quantitative methods expert, and one of the founders of the University of Pittsburgh's Pain Evaluation and Treatment Institute, has been a guiding beacon in my attention to detail and scientific thought process. Dr. Ronald Glick, a physiatrist at Pitt, initially inspired me to become an acupuncturist and changed the way I think about chronic pain.

The many patients with chronic low back pain for whom I have cared over the years and the participants in my research studies on chronic low back pain are truly the heart and soul of this book. While their stories have been included, the magnitude of their impact on me cannot be gleaned from the material that you are about to read. Chronic low back pain is extremely complex and poorly understood by the medical community. The patients for whom I have cared, however, understand it all too well, and through their understanding they have taught me about the aspects of this condition that are truly important.

Although I find the practice of medicine extremely rewarding, it is my wonderful family that gives my life depth and perspective. To my husband, Neal, and my children, Marc, Abby, and Rachel, thank you for giving me what no scholarly pursuit possibly could. Among my life's accomplishments, you are the pinnacle.

Contents

Introduction

———— ✒ ————

Because you've picked up this book, I am assuming you're a member of a not-so-exclusive "club," one of the millions of Americans who is needlessly suffering with chronic low back pain. Indeed, one reason I focus on low back pain in this book is that when we consider back pain in general, the vast majority of cases involve the lower spine rather than the upper or middle back, for reasons I address in great detail later in this book. Even more important, however, is a second reason: I believe Americans are suffering needlessly from this condition. I say this because my experience has shown me that if you are like most of the men and women in this category, you may not be benefiting from the many different integrative treatment options that can provide relief from your pain and disability. Why? Because these options were never offered or explained to you.

Instead, you and countless others probably have never undergone a thorough, comprehensive evaluation of your back pain. Whatever assessment you did experience was then likely followed by your being handed prescriptions for painkillers, sedatives, antidepressants, or muscle relaxants, and maybe a verbal reminder to do some back exercises and to "be careful." You were led to believe that a combination of pharmaceuticals and tentative living would need to become a permanent part of your life if you want to control your pain or prevent recurring episodes. In your mind, you may half believe you will never get significant relief, while the other half of you may be desperately holding out hope that you will.

I believe you *can* get relief. My experience has shown me that relief not only *is* possible, but that significant relief can often be achieved with minimal or no medications and the bothersome side effects all too often associated with them. I've found this to be true in people of all ages and from all walks of life, people who have wanted to take control of their back pain and their lives using techniques they have integrated into their lifestyles. So I wrote this book for you—thanks to them—to share with you how you can get relief, too.

Chronic back pain is a universal problem that crosses all age, ethnic, social, religious, and economic barriers. It has been called "the most expensive benign condition in industrialized countries," costing about $100 billion per year in the United States: 20 percent of that in direct, medically related costs and 80 percent in lost productivity. In the United States, low back pain is second only to the common cold as a cause for lost work time. Every year, 3 to 4 percent of the population is temporarily disabled by back pain, and 1 percent of working-age individuals are completely disabled by it. Low back pain accounts for 19 percent of all workers' compensation claims made in the United States. Among older adults, each year about 30 percent of those living outside institutions experience an episode of lower back pain, and 20 percent of them live with chronic pain.

So what can you do about chronic low back pain? Plenty. And you can begin by fortifying yourself with knowledge of your condition so you are better able to take back control of your life. To help you with that task, I wrote this book, in which I share my experiences and those of some of my patients at the University of Pittsburgh, where I am an internist, rheumatologist, geriatrician, and acupuncturist. I am also an associate professor of medicine, psychiatry, and anesthesiology, and director of the Older Adult Pain Management Program at the Pain Evaluation and Treatment Institute. In part I, I explain the facets of chronic back pain and its many contributing causes. Equally important, I discuss the importance of undergoing a comprehensive physical examination and personal evaluation and how you can help your physician make an accurate diagnosis. I also reveal why expensive, time-consuming tests, including X-rays and other imaging studies ordered by many doctors, often are not necessary and in fact may be misleading.

Then in part II, I explain my six-step approach to treatment. Several things are important to know about these therapeutic methods. First, five of them do *not* include surgical procedures. I believe back surgery should be reserved for individuals who either have not responded to other aggressive measures or whose physical function and/or quality of life is significantly and seriously impaired without it. Second, if a patient's treatment plan for chronic low back pain includes medication, it must also include several nonpharmacological approaches, such as percutaneous electrical nerve stimulation (PENS), Pilates, yoga, self-hypnosis, or meditation. I firmly believe that medication should be viewed as a means to an end, that is, a tool for rehabilitation and recovery, not an end in and of itself. Certainly, many of my patients have had either no need for that tool or much less of a need once they were properly diagnosed and a treatment plan had been put together for them.

Third, the order of the six steps is important in that the initial step should be undertaken first by virtually all patients except those who have a critical condition that requires them to proceed directly to step six, surgical intervention, the option of last resort. The therapy approaches in steps two through five can be incorporated into your treatment program along with your exercise plan, as you and your health-care practitioner see fit. You might view the process like a menu: you develop your main entrée—an exercise program—and add side dishes to complement it. Thus, one person's exercise plan may be enhanced by a monthly massage and self-hypnosis sessions, another may need to include an anti-inflammatory medication and administration of an epidural injection during the initial weeks of physical therapy to get started, while yet another may incorporate periodic chiropractic sessions and biofeedback.

It all comes down to this: it's important to educate yourself about your back and to be proactive in the development and implementation of your treatment and prevention program. This book explains the many options you have at your disposal to help you accomplish that goal and take back control of your life.

That's enough by way of introduction. Now let's get to work.

Part I

━━━━━━━━ ⌒✥⌒ ━━━━━━━━

UNDERSTANDING BACK PAIN

It's not as common as the common cold, but it's close: According to the National Institute of Neurological Disorders and Stroke, low back pain affects 70 to 85 percent of adults in the United States at some period in their lives. It is the most common cause of disability among people younger than forty-five, and it is a universal problem that crosses all age, ethnic, social, and economic barriers. Besides impacting the lives of millions of people every day, chronic low back pain and the common cold share another characteristic: we have not yet found a cure.

But what we *do* have is an arsenal of treatment techniques that are all too often ignored by physicians, who tend to favor writing prescriptions for painkillers or, a much more serious scenario, recommending surgery as the answer to chronic low back pain. My experience has shown me that the most effective way to treat this painful condition is through *a multidisciplinary approach that may require minimal or no medications.* This includes an exercise program, a variety of movement therapies, mind-body techniques, and lifestyle adjustments, with integration of medications if and when needed.

What exactly *is* chronic low back pain and where can you turn for help? In these first two chapters, I explain what we know about this painful condition, because I believe it's important for you to understand your back so you can more fully participate in healing it. Thus, I talk about various causes of back pain, how they are diagnosed, and how you can find knowledgeable professionals to help you get an accurate diagnosis and an effective treatment program.

Chapter 1

Your Aching Back: Why You Hurt

It's pretty basic: Before you can find effective, safe, long-lasting relief for your chronic back pain, it helps to know why you hurt. Once you have a handle on the cause of your pain, you can begin to review and implement the various approaches described in this book to help alleviate it. I also believe that you should have some knowledge of how to recognize the different conditions that may be causing your back pain and, more important, how to explain your pain and any accompanying symptoms. In this way, you can help your health-care practitioner arrive at a more accurate diagnosis. Also, I find that patients are more likely to stick with and follow a treatment program if they understand what they are treating and why. So let's get started with a few basics and then move on to the causes of your pain.

I introduce quite a few terms in this chapter and in the next one and a few illustrations to help you understand them better. Although it isn't critical for you to fully comprehend each of these

3

terms, I believe it's important that you are at least familiar with them, as they are words your doctors and physical therapists may use when they talk about your condition. And while the workings of the human body can seem truly amazing at times, I don't believe patients should be kept in the dark or mystified by what is happening to them, especially when they are in pain.

ACUTE VS. CHRONIC BACK PAIN

Acute or chronic? Acute pain is typically defined as pain that lasts less than three months, while a label of chronic indicates pain that lasts longer. In most cases, acute back pain is the result of a bodily injury, such as a muscle strain, that heals within a month or two. Often, however, chronic back pain begins as acute back pain that becomes persistent: there may be an acute physical injury that may be the result of an automobile accident or something as simple as straining a muscle while bending to pick up a pencil that has fallen onto the floor. Some patients who come to see me don't remember doing anything that triggered the pain. "It seemed to come out of nowhere," some tell me, or "It seems like I've been living with this back pain for so long, I can't even remember when it first started."

Symptoms of chronic low back pain vary. The pain may be stabbing, piercing, shooting, or throbbing; it may be localized or referred from another part of your body; it may occur only when you sit, stand, walk, or turn. Along with the chronic back pain, you may have other symptoms, such as fever, headache, tingling or pins and needles in your legs, muscle weakness, or weight loss—any one or more of which suggest you may have an infection or another medical condition that may be causing or contributing to your pain and should prompt you to seek immediate medical attention. One common symptom I see in patients who have chronic low back pain is depression, which is three to four times as prevalent in such patients as in the general population.

The Pain Paradox

A paradox about low back pain is that the severity of a person's physical condition does not necessarily translate into a similar level of pain. Some people, for example, have herniated discs, yet experience absolutely no pain, while other individuals can have a simple muscle sprain and become incapacitated. For some people, the pain flares up at irregular intervals, with weeks, months, and even years between episodes. Each episode can differ in severity, duration, and how it responds to treatment.

The important thing to remember is that all of these symptoms, and any I have not listed, as well as patterns of painful episodes are important to share with your health-care practitioner. Every bit of information is a piece of the puzzle, clues to the cause of your pain. Ultimately, they can help your physician determine the type of treatment options that will work best for you.

LOWER BACK BASICS

The spine is composed of up to thirty-three interlocking bones called vertebrae that are stacked in an S-shaped curve arrangement. This arrangement allows the spine to absorb the stress that body movement places on it, as well as helps it support the body's weight. These functions of the spine are not shared equally by the three regions that make up this structure, however (see figure 1.1). The vertebrae in the lower, or lumbar, region are thicker and sturdier than those above it, and for good reason: unlike the cervical and thoracic regions above it, the lumbar region performs the critical task of acting as a cushion for the weight of the upper body.

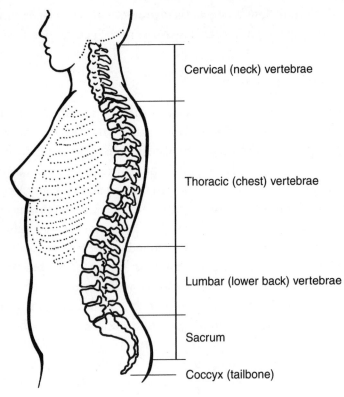

Cervical (neck) vertebrae

Thoracic (chest) vertebrae

Lumbar (lower back) vertebrae

Sacrum

Coccyx (tailbone)

Figure 1.1 The spinal column

The bottom of the lumbar region ends at the sacrum, a bone that consists of five vertebrae that are fused together. The sacrum, together with the pelvic bones, forms the pelvic girdle, a critical structure when it comes to the functioning of the spine, because it balances the spine and connects it with the legs.

The lumbar region is composed of a complicated infrastructure of nerves, muscles, tendons, ligaments, veins and arteries, vertebrae, and spongy cartilage tissue. While all of these structures contribute to the complexity of the lower back, the nerve supply is especially intricate, because much of it overlaps as it makes its way to the different muscles, ligaments, tendons, discs, and other tissues in the spine and legs. In fact, this overlap can make it very difficult for the brain to distinguish between an injury to, say, a disc versus a tendon.

For example, a herniated disc can feel just like an injured ligament or a bruised muscle, but it's important to differentiate them because they should be treated differently. Therefore, it's important for your physician to conduct a thorough medical history and physical examination, as well as get a detailed account from you about your symptoms. This is why I urge you to take notes—literally write down the information in a pocket-size notebook if you need to—about what you feel, when you feel it, and how long it lasts. Such input is key to the diagnostic process, which we will discuss in the next chapter.

Muscling In

If you get nothing else from this chapter, it's important to understand this about back pain and your muscles: If you want to win against chronic low back pain, you must keep your muscles healthy. The back consists of dozens of different muscles, and all of them work together, either directly or indirectly, and are connected to nearly every major muscle group in the body. Thus, when any muscle within this interconnected structure is stressed, tense, or in spasm, it can impact the function and health of many others throughout the body as well. Therefore, keeping your back muscles healthy is good for more than just your back; it benefits your entire body.

The significance of this connection is even more relevant once you know that muscle pain from a strain in your back is generally ten to twenty times more painful than a muscle strain that occurs anywhere else in the body. That's because most of the pain receptors in your back are in the muscles. Most people don't realize this fact, so when they experience back pain, they automatically think, "I must have a ruptured disc" or "I have a pinched nerve," when in most cases their muscles are causing the pain. And the pain does not have to feel like an ache; it can also be stabbing, piercing, burning, or throbbing.

That being said, let's take a quick look at some of the main muscles involved in keeping the lower back healthy. It may seem like I'm overwhelming you with a lot of terms, but I think it's important for you to have at least a casual knowledge of these muscles so you can get a better appreciation of the complexities of chronic low back pain. Plus, you may recognize some of the terms your health-care practitioners use when they talk to you.

First, let's talk about the muscles that support the spine. *Extensors* are a group of muscles that straighten the back as well as lift, extend, and move the thighs away from the body. Among this group is the largest muscle in the body—the gluteus maximus in your buttocks—which stabilizes the hips. It also attaches to the lumbodorsal fascia (a fascia is a fibrous, strong tissue that covers and/or separates muscles into groups), a structure that stabilizes the lumbar spine and pelvis and also works in conjunction with other pelvic and leg muscles. If your gluteus maximus is weak, you likely stand with your pelvis tilted one way or another, which places excessive stress on your hip capsules and lumbopelvic ligaments and allows your muscles to weaken. A weak gluteus maximus also permits more stress to be placed on your spinal discs and facets, which causes your lumbosacral joint (where the bottom of the lumbar spine, L5, meets the sacrum) to break down prematurely and contributes to low back pain. Another contributing factor is weak lower extremities. The weaker your leg muscles, the greater your tendency to depend on and eventually wear down your lumbar spine.

Another muscle group is the *flexors*—the abdominal and psoas muscles—which help bend and support the spine from the front of the body. They also flex and move the thigh in toward the body and influence the arch of the lower spine. Weak abdominal muscles are an invitation for lower back problems. When abdominal muscles are toned and strengthened, back pain often is reduced. (We'll talk much more about this in chapter 3.) The psoas muscles, which connect the bones of the upper thighs to the spine, support and stabilize the spinal column. Some people who experience severe back strain also report having pain on both sides of the groin. This pain may be caused by spasm of the psoas muscles, which react this way in an attempt to stabilize the spinal column.

The third group is the *obliques*, or rotator muscles (side muscles). These flat muscles stabilize the spine when you are upright, help stabilize and support the lower back and pelvis, rotate the spine and maintain correct posture and spinal curvature, and share some of the weight load with the discs, thus protecting them from injury.

Let's not forget the *hamstring muscles*, which are located in the back of the thigh. These muscles connect to the bottom of the pelvic bone, which connects to the base of the spine. If your hamstring muscles are tight—which is very common in people who sit a lot—a domino effect can occur: Tight hamstring muscles place stress on the pelvic bone, which pulls on the spine and transfers the weight of the spine onto the discs.

This creates instability in the spine and can lead to muscle spasms and tension on the spine. This is why it's important to stand up and stretch your hamstring muscles at least every few hours whenever you sit for a prolonged period. Hamstring muscles can also become tight from poor posture, especially swayback, which is characterized by an increase in the natural inward curve of the lower back.

If you have pain in your buttocks that travels down your leg, you may be feeling your *piriformis muscle*, which is located deep in the buttocks. If this muscle becomes constricted or spasms, it can irritate the sciatic nerve and cause the characteristic buttocks and back-of-the-leg pain associated with sciatica. We'll talk more about sciatica later.

Before we leave the muscles, I need to mention a few more structures that you'll read about in the next chapter: the *tensor fascia lata* and the *iliotibial band*. The tensor fascia lata is a short muscle, and the iliotibial band is fascia. As a unit, these structures run the length of the outer thigh. Individually, the tensor fascia lata flexes and internally rotates the hips, while both structures work together to help stabilize the leg while standing and are often involved, either directly or indirectly, with low back pain.

Intervertebral Discs

Perhaps the most talked about parts of the back are the discs or, more accurately, the intervertebral discs. These structures are formed from cartilaginous tissue and are sandwiched between and cushion each of the vertebrae, which prevents them from grinding against each other. The discs perform a critical role, as they help absorb shocks to the spinal column that are placed on it during everyday activities. In addition to handling the weight of the upper body, the lumbar region also must support the weight of whatever you pick up or carry, and your waist acts like the fulcrum, or pivoting point, in a lever system when you lift.

For example, if you lift a 10-pound bag of dog food, you place approximately 100 pounds of pressure on your lower back and increase the pressure inside your lumbar discs. This is a significant burden for your lumbar spine to bear. Intervertebral discs are designed to transmit and distribute that pressure evenly and thus allow normal activities to continue while preventing injuries. One reason discs are able to do this is their high water content makes them very elastic, which helps make and keep the spine flexible. For the first thirty or so years of life, the gel in the inner part of the disc (the nucleus pulposus) is composed of approximately 90 percent water. This percentage gradually decreases over the next forty years or so to about 65 percent. As the percentage decreases and the discs lose their thickness, the space between the facet joints also decreases. The overall result is a loss of disc height (and the related loss in skeletal height; we shrink as we age), reduced ability of the discs to absorb shock, and reduced flexibility, all reasons why the backs of older adults are less nimble than those of younger people.

Facet Joints

Another thing you'll hear quite a bit about is *facet joints*. Facet joints are paired, thumbnail-size joints located on the back of the spine, where they help stabilize the lower back and guide its motion. Each vertebra has an upper and lower facet that link together to form a joint. In some individuals, these joints become painful and stiff. We'll talk more about facet joint pain and how it can be diagnosed and treated in chapter 6.

All together, the structures of the lumbar region help to regulate the functions and impact the health of the abdominal and pelvic organs and muscles, as well as the bones and joints of the legs. Thus, the lower back is very vulnerable to stress, strain, sprains, and other injuries that may come its way, and the result of such injuries is often inflammation and pain.

Spinal Ligaments

The spinal ligaments have been likened to very tough rubber bands in that they are strong, elastic, and fibrous. These essential qualities allow them to perform their job, which is to help support the vertebrae and protect the spinal column from injury.

CAUSES OF LOW BACK PAIN

Lots of words get bandied about when people talk about low back pain, words that can be pretty scary. "Slipped disc," "bulging disc," "herniated disc," and "degenerative disc" are popular, as are phrases like "arthritis of the spine" and "scoliosis," or "curvature of the spine." And many people believe that these or other physical defects or weaknesses are the cause of their back pain. Fortunately, it's often just not true. (See Delia's Story below.)

The truth is, the majority of low back pain—about 97 percent—is caused by stress, trauma, or injury to the spine's muscles, ligaments, facets, or sacroiliac (SI) joint (more on these structures below). *Most chronic low back pain is muscle related.* Of that 97 percent, more than 70 percent is associated with muscle-related factors, such as strains, muscle tension and inflammation in the lumbar region, myofascial pain syndrome, and fibromyalgia, with degenerative disc or facet disease coming in a distant second (an estimated 10 percent). The remaining mechanical causes of low back pain are divided among various other physical conditions, which total about 14 percent. The remaining 3 percent is divided among diseases that affect different organ systems (about 2 percent) and nonmechanical spinal conditions (about 1 percent). (See the Causes of Low Back Pain table.)

Causes of Low Back Pain

Cause Category	Examples
Mechanical Conditions of the Spine (97%)	Muscle-related factors (e.g., strains, spasm, myofascial pain syndrome, fibromyalgia) (>70%).
	Degeneration of disc or facet (>10%)
	Compression fracture due to osteoporosis (4%)
	Herniated disc (4%)
	Spinal stenosis (3%)
	Spondylolisthesis (2%)
	Fracture due to trauma (<1%)
	Congenital disease, e.g., kyphosis, lordosis, scoliosis (<1%)
Diseases of Various Organ Systems (2%)	chronic pelvic inflammatory disease
	endometriosis
	kidney stones
	pyelonephritis (bacterial infection of the kidney)
	abdominal aortic aneurysm (a ballooning of the wall of the aorta)
	pancreatitis (inflammation of the pancreas)
	penetrating ulcer
Nonmechanical Conditions of the Spine (1%)	Paget's disease
	inflammatory arthritis
	neoplasia
	infection

That being said, I want to point out that these figures take into account people of all ages. Therefore, the balance of the figures changes somewhat when we look at a specific population, such as people sixty years and older, who are less likely to experience sprains and strains and herniated discs, but who have a greater tendency to experience degenerative processes of discs and facets, compression fractures, spinal stenosis, and fractures due to trauma (especially falls). One thing that does not change when we factor in age, however, is that *chronic low back pain very often has muscle-related causes.*

Another point I want to make is that while many people say their back pain seemed to "come out of nowhere," in most cases it is a manifestation of an accumulated series of conditions and events, including aging, a history of weak abdominal and back muscles, poor posture, obesity, and incorrect lifting and carrying habits. So although it may seem like your back pain suddenly appeared when you bent down to tie your shoes or put your groceries into the trunk of your car, such isolated activities were more likely, if you'll forgive me, the last straw.

Delia's Story

Delia, a sixty-five-year-old retired school administrator, came to see me complaining of severe pain that she described as "like someone is sticking a hot poker into my left buttock." Other complaints included depression, difficulty sleeping, and most distressing to her, an inability to continue ballroom dancing, an activity she had been teaching at her local senior center and in which she had participated for pleasure and competition for many years. She had had the pain fairly constantly for more than eight months and had been diagnosed by her primary-care physician as having osteoarthritis, for which he had prescribed nonsteroidal anti-inflammatory drugs (NSAIDs). The drugs provided minimal relief, and Delia was very upset about not being able to resume dancing.

During my physical examination of Delia, I noted severe tenderness of the left piriformis, a muscle that lies deep in the buttocks and travels from the base of the spine and attaches to the thigh bone near the outside crease of the buttock. Although Delia had complained of this pain previously to two other doctors, neither one had done a hands-on examination and both had incorrectly diagnosed her as having osteoarthritis. Clearly, piriformis myofascial pain was the source of Delia's "poker" pain. I prescribed physical therapy, but her insurance carrier refused to pay for noninvasive treatment for her "same problem." In fact, Delia had been treated for osteoarthritis, not piriformis pain, but although she explained to the insurance company that she was not being treated for the "same problem," she was unsuccessful in getting coverage for the physical therapy. Physical therapy was the treatment option Delia and I preferred, but because she was limited by finances, I ordered a series of injections of the piriformis and discontinued the NSAIDs. Within a month, Delia was enjoying a significant reduction in her pain, restful sleep every night, and a return to ballroom dance, both in the classroom and on the dance floor.

If Delia had been diagnosed accurately when she first sought medical help, she could have avoided months of pain and continued to participate in activities that meant much to her and enhanced her quality of life. She also could have avoided the use of NSAIDs and the side effects that accompany them.

Muscle-Related Pain

As I've already mentioned, the vast majority of persistent lower back pain is associated with some type of trauma or other factor that affects the muscles. In this category, we're looking at several contributors.

- **Strain** refers to the overstretching or overexertion of a muscle.
- **Spasm** is the sudden, involuntary contraction of a muscle or group of muscles in response to trauma that has occurred in a muscle, disc, joint, or ligament.
- **Myofascial pain** is a type of pain that affects the muscles and can cause local or referred pain, tenderness, stiffness and limited movement, muscle weakness, and tightness. Although most people think of muscle pain as being an aching sensation, myofascial pain can also be experienced as stabbing or burning.
- **Fibromyalgia** is a condition characterized by widespread chronic pain that people experience in muscles, but the muscles themselves are not abnormal or damaged. The problem in this condition seems to be an inability of the central nervous system to process pain normally.

While it is true that muscle strains and spasms are usually associated with acute low back pain, in some cases they may also trigger other processes that ultimately result in chronic pain. In fact, the transition from acute pain to chronic pain may be caused by various neurophysiological, psychological, social, and other factors about which the individual in pain may not be aware.

From Acute Pain to Chronic Pain

On a neurophysiological level, for example, an acute injury may trigger a latent painful condition (see Myofascial Pain Syndrome below) or sensitize certain nerve cells so that they react in an exaggerated way to stimulation. A strain or spasm could also alter the way nerve cells send out their signals, resulting in an abnormal response to stimuli. Damaged tissues may also release substances that change a person's perception of pain. None of this means that the pain you feel isn't real or is "only in your head." But it *does* suggest that you have some control over your pain, which I explain in part II of this book.

Psychologically, the presence of pain can be very stressful. Many people adopt "pain behavior," meaning they restrict their movements and activities, sometimes to the point of spending days or even weeks in bed. Why? Patients say they are "afraid" to exercise because they might hurt themselves further. Fear of the unknown, of not knowing if or when the pain will go away or of moving in a way that will send more waves of pain through their back, severely restricts the activities of some people. A significant reduction in movement or exercise, however, quickly results in a loss of muscle strength and tone and can ultimately make movement more painful, perhaps even leading to chronic pain. In people with chronic low back pain, for example, the lumbar extensor muscles are weaker than the lumbar flexor muscles. Chronic back pain also leads to a weakening of the multifidus and longissimus muscles, which are the muscles you use for lifting.

Patients may also talk about their pain to others, getting reinforcement for their behavior. The emotional stress caused by pain also increases activity in the sympathetic nervous system and increases the activity of norepinephrine (a chemical substance—neurotransmitter—in the brain whose elevated levels are associated with pain), which may further enhance a person's perception of pain. Often, people in pain become anxious and/or depressed and may become worried about their ability to continue working, caring for and providing financially for their family, and enjoying activities in which they participated in the past. Anxiety, depression, and fear can result in people feeling hopeless and helpless, with no control over their lives. These feelings have a negative effect on people's motivation to seek treatment and/or comply with their doctor's treatment plan.

Clearly, the evolution of chronic low back pain is not simple. Any one or more of these and other factors can be involved in the process, and an experienced diagnostician will explore the physical, psychological, social, and environmental factors that may have contributed to a person's chronic pain. (We'll look at the diagnostic process in chapter 2.) Now, however, I want to talk about two syndromes that are often overlooked as muscle-related causes of chronic low back pain: myofascial pain syndrome and fibromyalgia syndrome.

Myofascial Pain Syndrome. My experience has shown me that myofascial pain is a major contributor to chronic low back pain and, unfortunately, a diagnosis many physicians do not explore. It is my hope that this will change, because I believe that taking the time to consider this diagnosis will result in a great many people receiving appropriate and effective treatment that may reduce their pain and significantly improve their lifestyle, often with little or no need for medications. Myofascial pain syndrome is a chronic musculoskeletal pain disorder that affects the fascia, the connective tissue that covers the muscles. It may involve a single muscle or a muscle group. Myofascial pain syndrome can develop from a muscle injury or lesion, or from excessive strain on a specific muscle or muscle group. It can also result from irritation of the nerves that feed the muscles, such as pressure on a spinal nerve root related to spinal arthritis. The irritated muscle that results then develops a *trigger point*, which causes pain that can be burning, stabbing, throbbing, and debilitating.

In fact, one of the classic signs of myofascial pain is trigger points, very tender sites within a taut band in a muscle. There are several types of trigger points, which I discuss in the next chapter on diagnosis. Here I want to emphasize that taut bands and trigger points are believed to be common in the general population and that millions of people may have the "makings" of low back pain associated with myofascial pain. That means it's important for physicians to be aware of and know how to recognize this syndrome.

Overall, the good news about myofascial pain syndrome is that there are many nonsurgical and nonpharmaceutical approaches you can explore to get relief from your pain. In fact, myofascial pain syndrome is most effectively treated with such approaches as specialized massage (trigger-point therapy), acupuncture, and/or trigger-point injections. We discuss them in detail in part II.

Fibromyalgia. Fibromyalgia is a syndrome characterized by chronic pain, including back pain, as well as stiffness and tenderness of muscles, tendons, ligaments, and joints without detectable inflammation. Fibromyalgia is also associated with other significant symptoms, which I discuss in the next chapter, all of which can have a devastating impact on people's abilities to go about their daily activities. The syndrome affects women more than men (>80 percent) and usually first appears during middle age.

Bonnie, a thirty-eight-year-old financial analyst, experienced firsthand the devastating effects of fibromyalgia. After spending months going to several different doctors and getting no answers or relief from her overwhelming fatigue, chronic back pain, sleep problems, and increasing muscle tenderness and stiffness, she went to one of my colleagues, who diagnosed her with fibromyalgia. By that time she had had to negotiate with her employer to reduce her workload and to allow her to work at home.

"I was fortunate that my boss allowed me to work at home, but I was so exhausted and in so much pain much of the time that even that was an effort," Bonnie explained. "With my back pain, I couldn't sit or stand for more than ten minutes at a time. My most comfortable position was on my side, curled up in a fetal position." My colleague consulted with me, and I prescribed a physical therapy program for Bonnie that included light stretching exercises to be done at home, massage, and water aerobics. Over the next few months, the program provided her with significant relief from both her back pain and her fatigue, and she was able to increase her workload and enjoy more restful sleep.

The exact underlying cause or causes of fibromyalgia are unknown, but continuing research is leading us to a better understanding of the condition. Most experts agree that fibromyalgia is a central nervous system disorder, specifically involving abnormalities in neuroendocrine and neurotransmitter activity. (Thus, although I listed fibromyalgia under "muscle-related causes" of chronic low back pain, it is at its core a nervous system disorder. Because of its profound impact on muscle, however, it is still appropriate to include it in this category.) In short, patients experience exaggerated, excessive pain due to abnormal processing of sensory signals by the central nervous system.

Fibromyalgia is diagnosed with a thorough history and physical examination. There are no definitive laboratory tests or X-rays to help with diagnosis. Patients with fibromyalgia also often suffer from myofascial pain syndrome. I discuss these two common conditions more thoroughly in chapter 2.

Degeneration of Discs and Facet Joints

Although it's common to believe that deterioration of the spine is limited to the elderly, the truth is that degeneration of the discs and facet joints in the lumbar spine can begin as early as adolescence and is common among people in their twenties. How quickly and to what degree the discs and joints wear out depends on several factors, not least of which are genetics; a person's weight; strength of the abdominal and back muscles; whether the individual smokes; and the type, amount, and manner of twisting, lifting, standing, sitting, and bending a person has done over the years. Depending on a person's activity choices and level, pressure on the lumbar spine can range from one to eleven times an individual's body weight.

Degeneration of the discs and facet joints in the lumbar spine is referred to as spinal osteoarthritis. This condition most often affects the lumbar spine in people who are older than forty and typically involves more than one vertebra. Several factors can contribute to degeneration of discs and facet joints. One is a reduction in the strength of the back muscles, which optimally share about one-third of the burden placed on the spine. This age-related loss places additional stress on the discs and facet joints.

Another significant factor, as mentioned previously, is the loss of water in intervertebral discs as people age. The reduction in water causes the discs to flatten and reduces the cushion between the vertebrae. In some people, a lifetime of stress on the lumbar spine causes some of the vertebrae to develop bone spurs (osteophytes), which can press on a spinal nerve and cause pain. Yet another factor is a deterioration of facet joints due to simple wear and tear, as well as loss of the cartilage that lines the facet joints due to arthritis.

Once again, a variety of nonsurgical, nonpharmaceutical options are available to effectively manage the pain and discomfort associated with degeneration of the discs and facet joints. We'll explore them in part II of this book.

Herniated Disc

"Whenever I hear the phrase 'herniated disc,' I wince," said Lydia, a forty-five-year-old marketing analyst who came to me believing she had a herniated disc (she did not). "The words alone sound painful." Yet although this condition sounds painful, experts have found that most people who have a herniated disc never experience symptoms. For those who do, however, the pain can vary from mild to severe; it may come and go or persist for weeks or months; and it can have a moderate to highly disruptive effect on their lives.

A herniated disc typically does not happen suddenly; it develops over time as the outer layer of the disc becomes thinner and weakens. Minute tears appear in the disc, while the water content at the center of the disc gradually decreases. This combination of factors makes the disc susceptible to herniation, in which the center of the disc protrudes through the weakened outer layer. Herniation can be triggered by a seemingly benign event, such as a sneeze or taking a jar of coffee out of the kitchen cabinets, or it may result from more serious trauma, such as an automobile accident or a fall. In 90 to 95 percent of cases, the herniation occurs in one or both of the lowest discs, L4-L5, and may affect the sacrum (L5-S1) as well.

The protruding disc can press on one or more spinal nerves or on the spinal cord itself or the cauda equina, the bundle of nerve roots located at the bottom of the spinal cord. Pressure on the nerves results in pain in other parts of the body as well as in the back. In most cases, a herniated disc does not require surgery, as it responds well to various physical and mind-body therapies, which I discuss in part II. The tissues that affect a herniated disc typically respond favorably as well to an epidural corticosteroid injection, which I discuss in chapter 6. Rarely, a herniated disc concentrates the compression on the cauda equina, causing individuals to lose nerve function in their bowels and bladder. Such conditions require immediate surgical intervention.

Although it usually takes time for a herniated disc itself to develop, the pain commonly occurs suddenly. "Something snapped," said Glenda, a thirty-four-year-old real estate agent who felt the pain of her herniated disc as she got out of her car at a client's house. "First I felt some tingling in my back, and it got worse and worse. Then I felt a snap and a terrible pain knifed through my back and left leg. I couldn't take a step, and the next thing I knew I was on the ground next to my car."

Some people who experience painful herniated discs have a history of athletic activity, such as football, gymnastics, dance, wrestling, track, diving, or hockey; others do not. Glenda had run track in college but had drifted away from running until about two years ago, when she began to jog several mornings a week. After her latest incident left her on the ground, she rethought her exercise program.

"The treatment I got for my herniated disc—exercise, acupuncture, massage—taught me a whole new appreciation for my body and what it can do," said Glenda. "I never want to feel that kind of pain again or feel so helpless, so I decided to take care of my back and to have fun doing it. My physical therapist suggested tai chi, yoga, and Pilates. I tried all three and stuck with the first two. I really enjoy them and believe they are keeping my back in shape."

The vast majority of herniated discs respond very well to treatment and heal well using a combination of exercise, physical therapy, and mind-body therapies over a period of two to three months or, if appropriate, injection therapy, which can result in much faster relief. I discuss these treatments in depth in part II.

Vertebral Compression Fracture

In healthy individuals, the vertebrae can withstand the pressures of everyday life and break only if subjected to some form of trauma, such as an automobile accident, a blow to the back, or a serious fall. But in individuals whose bone density—specifically of their spine—is compromised and weakened by conditions such as osteoporosis, Paget's disease, hyperparathyroidism, or cancer, something as simple as a cough or sneeze can cause a compression fracture (i.e., collapse) of a vertebra.

Vertebral compression fractures occur most often in the middle to lower back, and the pain associated with such fractures tends to correspond with the injured area and worsen when the individual sits or stands. Some people also experience thigh, abdominal, or hip pain. Weakness, tingling, or numbness of a leg suggests compression of the nerves at the fracture site, while an inability to urinate or loss of control of the bowels indicates that the fracture is pressing on the spinal cord. People who have several vertebral compression fractures may lose height and have a rounded back, a condition that is sometimes called kyphosis (a dowager's hump).

By far the most common cause of vertebral compression fractures is osteoporosis, with approximately seventy thousand people a year experiencing such fractures. When a compression fracture is caused by osteoporosis, the fracture usually occurs in the front of the vertebra, which causes the bone in front of the spine to collapse and leaves the back of the same bone still intact. The result is a wedge-shaped vertebra and a fracture that is stable and often painless. In rare cases, there is nerve or spinal cord damage.

It has been estimated that 25 percent of American women fifty years and older have one or more compression fractures, and the number rises to 40 percent among women eighty years and older. Such fractures affect about 14 percent of older men. Therefore, the possibility of a vertebral compression fracture should be considered in older adults who complain of chronic low back pain and who have one or more of the symptoms mentioned above, especially among women. I want to emphasize, however, that because many vertebral compression fractures due to osteoporosis are asymptomatic, I encourage especially women to take preventive measures against osteoporosis and to get screened every few years, beginning around age forty. (See the resources section for sources of information on osteoporosis prevention.)

One thing that makes vertebral compression fractures associated with osteoporosis of great concern is the list of complications that often accompany them. Constipation, deep venous thrombosis, loss of independence, prolonged pain and inactivity, bowel obstruction, pneumonia, progressive muscle weakness, crowding of internal organs, emotional problems, and loss of height often lead to individuals being unable to care for themselves, which frequently results in a need for nursing-home care. An accurate, prompt diagnosis and aggressive treatment can make it possible for more and more people to live relatively pain-free and to maintain their independence, issues of great concern as the number of older Americans keeps increasing.

Vertebral compression fractures are also found among people who have Paget's disease, which is most common among older adults. The disease is characterized by excessive development of unorganized bone, most notably in the spine, pelvis, and thigh, that is inherently weak and highly susceptible to fracture. In hyperparathyroidism, the parathyroid gland produces excessive parathyroid hormone, which promotes calcium loss from bone and stimulates the activity of osteoclasts, cells that break down bone. Cancer that has spread to the spine can also cause vertebral compression fractures. Cancers most often associated with this problem are prostate, breast, and multiple myeloma.

Treatment of vertebral compression fractures involves addressing both the back pain and the contributing factor, which in most cases is osteoporosis. A variety of treatment options for the back pain are discussed in part II.

Spinal Stenosis

In a small percentage of people, the spinal canal becomes narrow due to degenerative changes in the spine that occur with wear and tear and age, a complication of surgery, Paget's disease, or trauma to the spine. Narrowing of the spinal canal, or *spinal stenosis*, usually starts slowly and causes pain not only in the back but also in the buttocks and both legs. The pain is often described as dull or aching and may be accompanied by numbness, tingling, or a loss of strength in the legs. One of the dangers of spinal stenosis is that the weakness in the legs makes people with this condition susceptible to falls. Another danger is that spinal stenosis may cause urinary incontinence if pressure is placed on the nerves that control the bladder. Spinal stenosis most often affects people in their fifties and sixties and is about twice as common in men as in women. Based on magnetic resonance imaging (MRI) findings, more than 20 percent of older adults may have spinal stenosis, although they are just as likely as not to have pain from the abnormality.

The pain of spinal stenosis is similar to that of intermittent claudication, a condition characterized by blocked blood flow to the legs. In chapter 2, I talk about how to identify spinal stenosis, and then in part II, I discuss the options available for treatment of spinal stenosis, including but not limited to physical therapy, epidural injections, acupuncture, movement therapies, and in a limited number of cases, a lumbar brace.

Spondylolysis and Spondylolisthesis

These two disorders account for about 2 percent of low back pain cases. Spondylolysis is the term for a stress fracture in a vertebra, most often the fifth lumbar (L5) vertebra and much less often the fourth lumbar vertebra (L4). It also refers to microtrauma of the bone that connects the facets (called the pars interarticularis), a condition often seen in adolescent athletes; or it can be a congenital defect or other bone disorder. If the stress fracture weakens the vertebra to a point where it no longer can maintain its correct position, the vertebra can begin to shift. The result can be spondylolisthesis, a term formed from two Greeks words: *spondylos*, which means "vertebra," and *olisthēsis*, which means "to slide on an incline." Thus, spondylolisthesis can be described as a disorder in which one vertebra slips over one below it. Spondylolisthesis can also occur without spondylolysis; for example, when a facet degenerates. The most common site for spondylolisthesis to occur is in the lumbar spine, specifically L4 and L5, where it is associated with low back pain, thigh or leg pain, muscle spasms, weakness, and/or tight hamstring muscles.

Like many other back disorders, spondylolysis and spondylolisthesis do not cause any symptoms in some individuals, even though their spinal X-rays clearly show they have these spinal abnormalities. Both conditions can be congenital (present at birth) or can develop anytime thereafter. In fact, some individuals are born with thin vertebrae and are therefore susceptible to spondylolysis and spondylolisthesis, especially if they participate in such activities as football, wrestling, dancing, gymnastics, or weightlifting during their growth years. Spondylolysis and spondylolisthesis also can develop due to other physical stresses to the spine, such as carrying heavy items, trauma from an accident, and general wear and tear.

Degenerative spondylolisthesis occurs most often after age forty and is seen more frequently with increasing age. Women are affected about five times more often than are men. It is also more common among people who have diabetes.

Fortunately, spondylolysis and spondylolisthesis can be treated successfully using the nonsurgical and nonpharmaceutical options discussed in part II of this book. Surgery could be necessary, however, in those very rare cases of spondylolisthesis in which the vertebrae press on nerve roots and cause the legs to become numb or weak.

Other Mechanical Causes of Low Back Pain

About 1 percent of chronic low back pain is attributed to fractures due to trauma (e.g., an automobile accident or a serious fall) or to congenital disease, such as kyphosis, lordosis, and scoliosis. Briefly, *kyphosis* is characterized by abnormal flexion (bending forward) of the spine. Although kyphosis is more common in the thoracic spine, it does appear in the lumbar region as well. Among adults, causes of kyphosis include trauma to the spine, including the effects of surgery or other medical treatment; congenital malformations (present from birth), in which development of the spine was abnormal; and osteoporosis, which is the most common cause among adults. Older women are more prone to kyphosis than are men or younger women.

A condition known as postural kyphosis, or "round back," is typically seen in adolescents and young adults and is the result of poor posture. Unlike "real" kyphosis, in which there is structural damage or abnormalities, the spine of an individual who has postural kyphosis does not have deformities. Treatment for adult kyphosis includes physical therapy, movement therapies, and/or bracing, while postural kyphosis responds to posture retraining, such as Feldenkrais (see chapter 3).

Lordosis, also known as swayback, is a condition in which there is increased curvature of the normally curved lumbar spine. The result is that the buttocks are thrust too far back and the abdomen is thrust too far forward. It is common among individuals who are overweight and have weak abdominal muscles. *Scoliosis* is a term used to describe an abnormal, side-to-side (lateral) curve in the spinal column that results in a sideways bend to the back. In the general population, about 2 percent of women and 0.5 percent of men are affected by this condition, which can vary greatly in severity. Among older adults (sixty years and older), however, studies indicate that the percentages are much greater—32 percent to as high as 68 percent, reported in a May 2005 study. Many of these cases involve mildly abnormal curvature and do not cause low back pain. Another age group greatly affected by scoliosis is adolescents. Idiopathic scoliosis (of unknown cause) develops in young adults around the beginning of puberty and affects about 500,000 adolescents in the United States. When chronic low back pain is associated with scoliosis, physical therapy and movement therapies can be effective (see chapter 3).

Organic and Nonmechanical Causes of Low Back Pain

About 2 percent of chronic low back pain can be attributed to referred pain from various organs in the abdominal and pelvic areas, such as the kidneys, stomach, intestines, and uterus. Some women, for example, experience referred back pain from endometriosis or pelvic inflammatory disease. Two other common sources of referred pain to the lower back include peptic ulcer disease and diverticulitis. Additional causes include pyelonephritis, abdominal aortic aneurysm, pancreatitis, and kidney stones.

In about 1 percent of cases, nonmechanical conditions of the spine are behind chronic back pain. Infections, such as osteomyelitis (infection of the vertebrae), abscesses inside the spine, Lyme disease, and varicella zoster virus (which causes shingles) are all possible sources, as are Paget's disease and inflammatory arthritis. Cancer that has spread to the spine, especially from breast or prostate cancer, as well as lymphoma and myeloma that invade the vertebrae, and benign tumors such as neurofibromas can cause back pain.

Yet One More Important Cause

I want to include a discussion of one more cause of back pain as an aside, because it is often overlooked by doctors and even suppressed by patients who don't want to "bother" their doctors with the complaint or who think nothing can be done about it. As a result, these individuals miss out on a better quality of life. The cause is back pain that develops as a result of surgery unrelated to the back; for example, hip surgery, hip replacement, or knee replacement. This type of back pain typically occurs in older adults and may be muscle-related. Stella's case is a good example.

Stella's Story

Stella had had arthritis in her right hip for about twenty years and had treated the pain with ibuprofen for much of that time, but by age seventy, the increasing pain and the deterioration in her hip led her to decide on hip replacement surgery. Up until that time, Stella had experienced what she called "the usual amount of low back pain"—brief, mild episodes throughout the years, but never anything that prevented her from working as an elementary school teacher or from gardening. "It was my hip that finally did me in," she said, "never my back."

But while she was recovering from successful hip surgery, she began to notice the beginnings of nagging lower back pain. She didn't mention it to her doctor or physical therapist because "I figured it would go away once I fully recovered from the surgery." She couldn't hide the pain from her therapist, however, who asked her if her back was troubling her, and she admitted that it was.

"My therapist explained that I had been compensating for my hurting hip for decades, and that part of my

compensation had kept me in a slightly forward position. Now that my hip is 'cured' and I can extend my hip
and leg in a normal way, muscles in my lower back that I
wasn't using much before are being used now, and so my
back hurts. That meant we had to make adjustments to
my exercise program to address those muscles. Once we
did that, the pain slowly began to improve."

Not all back pain that develops after a total joint replacement (e.g., hip, knee) is muscle-related. In some cases, individuals are left with a leg length discrepancy that can cause
sacroiliac joint pain that may require treatment with a shoe lift.

If you have had similar surgery not related to your back and
are now experiencing chronic low back pain, the changes in
your body alignment that resulted from your surgery could be
placing new stress on your low back muscles. Fortunately, you
can strengthen those muscles with the right physical therapy
and exercise. I recommend you talk to your physician and/or a
physical therapist so you can begin to make those changes
today and more fully enjoy the benefits of your surgery.

Stella's story introduces yet another factor to consider when
looking at causes of chronic low back pain. In some individuals, low back pain is a major characteristic of arthritis of the
hip, and so doctors and patients often focus on the back pain
and miss the diagnosis of arthritis. The result can be inappropriate and ineffective treatment. I talk more about hip arthritis and chronic back pain in chapter 2.

IN CONCLUSION . . .

By far, the most common causes of chronic low back pain are
mechanical—related to problems with, damage to, or abnor-

malities of the vertebrae and/or intervertebral discs, as well as specific muscles, ligaments, tendons, and nerves. That being said, it is important to rule out other possible causes of the pain, because a misdiagnosis and subsequent inappropriate treatment may result in prolonged pain, unnecessary suffering, and possibly greater damage to your health.

On that note, let's now turn to the diagnostic process. It is essential that you undergo a comprehensive examination and evaluation conducted by knowledgeable health-care professionals before you can be sure you are proceeding on the best treatment path for your needs. In the next chapter, we look at who those professionals are and how I believe back pain should be evaluated so an accurate diagnosis can be made.

Chapter 2

Getting Help for Your Chronic Back Pain

Back pain is so prevalent in our society, it's not unusual to hear people of all ages and from all walks of life and backgrounds say, "I've got a bad back" or "Sorry, I can't lift that, my back is bad." (Notice, however, that no one ever says, "I have a *good* back!") Over many years, I have diagnosed, treated, and come to know many of these individuals, and I have seen the toll chronic pain can take. For many men and women, chronic low back pain has a dramatic effect on their lives—physically, emotionally, mentally, socially, and financially. I have also observed that there is one thing these individuals share, in addition to pain: a strong desire and need to be heard, to have their pain validated, and to get relief. They deserve these things, and so do you. In this chapter, I explain how to accomplish these desires: which professionals you need to talk to, what you should tell them, and how I believe a comprehensive evaluation of chronic back pain should be conducted.

My job and that of my colleagues would be easier if the exact cause(s) of low back pain was more readily apparent. Yet several factors make diagnosis difficult. The complex structure of the back, which I discussed briefly in chapter 1, can make it challenging to find precisely why any given individual is experiencing chronic low back pain. Then there's another twist: many people who experience severe back and leg pain have no physical abnormalities to explain the pain, while many others have conditions normally associated with back pain, such as herniated discs, but are pain-free.

Yet one more factor must be considered: psychological impact. Because there is such a close relationship between the body and the mind, especially when it comes to the experience of pain, the cause of chronic back pain is rarely just physical. That's one reason I find the mind-body therapies (see chapters 4 and 5) to be so effective when treating chronic back pain. It is also why I believe that as part of the diagnostic process, it is necessary to look beyond the signs and symptoms that patients bring to the doctor's office and consider other important, contributing factors, such as the impact of emotional, financial, and social stressors and the presence of other medical conditions, such as arthritis, diabetes, osteoporosis, depression, and dementia. All of these factors can alter if and how a patient will comply with treatment recommendations, especially when it comes to a home exercise program or going to physical therapy. These factors also have an impact on how patients actually experience their pain, especially those who have dementia or who are depressed, which can influence how we treat such patients. Fortunately, we in the medical community have many tools to help us effectively and accurately evaluate low back pain, and I talk about them in this chapter.

Before we get into a discussion of the diagnostic process, however, I want to introduce the "we," the various professionals you need to consult and work with on your healing journey.

FINDING PROFESSIONAL HELP

"Who do I see to get relief for chronic back pain?" asked Christine, a thirty-eight-year-old mother of three and piano teacher. "We've got cardiologists for the heart, podiatrists for the feet, ophthalmologists for the eyes, gastroenterologists for the stomach, but who takes care of the back? Do I go to a rheumatologist, orthopedist, neurologist, general practitioner? What I need is a backtologist!"

First Stop: Primary Care

In today's health-care environment, which revolves largely around managed care, your first stop is likely to be your primary-care physician, who most likely falls into one of the following categories:

- **General Practitioners:** Physicians who are consulted for general health problems and do not specialize in a specific area of medicine. They can conduct an initial examination and prescribe tests and/or medications as appropriate or refer you to a specialist if they believe further testing or evaluation is needed. In terms of training, a general practitioner has completed a one-year internship following his or her completion of a four-year doctor of medicine (M.D.) or doctor of osteopathy (D.O.) degree.

- **Family Practitioners:** Physicians who are trained to care for patients of all ages. Like general practitioners, they too conduct examinations, prescribe medication, and make referrals. However, family practitioners have completed a three-year family medicine residency following their M.D. or D.O. degree.
- **Internists:** Physicians who specialize in the diagnosis and medical treatment of adults. Internists may have a subspecialty in one or more areas, such as rheumatology or geriatric medicine.
- **Osteopaths:** Physicians whose training parallels that of M.D.s (i.e., allopathic physicians) and is followed by four years in osteopathic college, where the emphasis is on the role of the musculoskeletal system (muscles, ligaments, tendons, bones) and the use of spinal manipulation.

Next Stop: A Specialist

Depending on your signs and symptoms, the results of any tests, and the availability of specialists in your area, your primary-care physician may then refer you to a specialist, such as one of the following:

- **Rheumatologists:** Internists who concentrate on treating the many different types of arthritis and related conditions, including fibromyalgia and osteoarthritis.
- **Orthopedists/Orthopedic Surgeons:** Specialists trained to treat diseases and injuries related to the musculoskeletal system. Orthopedic surgeons are trained in the diagnosis and treatment of spinal disorders, trauma, fractures, and arthritis. They, along with neurosurgeons,

are the physicians most likely to perform back surgeries. Each type of specialist, however, is specially trained to handle different types of back problems. For example, an orthopedic surgeon is better trained to do spine deformity surgery (e.g., scoliosis) than is a neurosurgeon, who would be more likely to do surgery for back tumors.

- **Neurologists/Neurosurgeons:** Physicians (M.D. or D.O.) who are trained in the diagnosis and treatment of disorders of the brain, nerves, spine, and the spinal cord and surrounding tissues. Neurologists focus on clinical examination, testing, and the use of medication for these disorders, but do not perform surgery. Neurosurgeons focus on the surgical treatment of patients who have these conditions.

- **Sports Medicine Specialists:** Physicians (M.D. or D.O.) who specialize in the treatment of musculoskeletal injuries, generally sports-related. More and more sports medicine specialists, though certainly not all, are including various integrative approaches, such as acupuncture, chiropractic, massage, and hydrotherapy, as part of their treatment plans.

- **Physiatrists:** Physicians who have specialized training in physical medicine and rehabilitation. Physiatrists do not perform surgery but instead prescribe therapies such as massage, biofeedback, traction, exercise, hot/cold therapy, transcutaneous electrical nerve stimulation (TENS), epidural spinal injections, and facet joint injections, as well as medications and braces. They work in hospitals, private practices, and rehabilitation centers.

- **Pain Medicine Specialists:** Physicians who have been

specially trained in the diagnosis and management of subacute and chronic pain, such as back pain, cancer, migraine, arthritis, and postsurgical pain. The American Board of Anesthesiology is the only organization recognized by the American Board of Medical Specialties that offers special credentials in pain medicine.

- **Anesthesiologists:** Physicians who manage pain both in and out of the operating room and who diagnose and treat both acute and chronic pain conditions.

- **Interventional Radiologists:** Physicians who have specialized in radiology and completed additional training in performing minimally invasive treatments using imaging techniques, such as X-rays, ultrasound, computerized axial tomography (CT), and MRI to guide very small surgical instruments through blood vessels or other pathways to detect or treat disease. These professionals frequently administer sacroiliac joint injections.

- **Physical Therapists:** Health professionals who are trained to provide services that help restore physical function, improve mobility, relieve pain, and prevent further or additional physical disabilities. Physical therapists test and measure patients' physical abilities, develop treatment plans that can include a wide range of therapies (e.g., from exercise to electrical stimulation to cold packs to massage), and teach patients to use assistive devices. Physical therapists typically work very closely with a patient's doctor and any other health-care professionals who are involved in a patient's care.

What You Should Know About Your Health-Care Practitioner

You can gather information about any health-care practitioner you plan to visit by questioning his or her office staff or by asking the practitioner directly. You are also entitled to see a copy of your doctor's resume. The office staff should provide this for you at your request.

- Professional degree held: medical physician (M.D.), doctor of osteopathy (D.O.), a Ph.D. in exercise physiology or nursing, a doctor of chiropractic (D.C.), and so on. You want to be sure the individual you choose for a specific service is qualified to provide it.

- Board certification: If applicable, what national board certification examination did he or she complete? There is a difference between board-eligible and board-certified. *Board-eligible* means the physician has completed the required training but has not yet passed the examination. *Board-certified* means the doctor has passed the examination. Board certifications are also awarded to other practitioners, including chiropractors, psychologists, and physical therapists. You can check any practitioner's board certification by contacting the organization that awards it (see the resources section). For example, for physicians, you can contact the American Board of Medical Specialties or the American Medical Association; for chiropractors, you can contact the American Chiropractic Association.

- Knowledge of back problems: Does the practitioner have specialized training in the diagnosis and/or treatment of low back pain?

- Conservative approach: Does the practitioner use a conservative (nonsurgical) approach? This question is important when dealing with specialists who may be trained primarily as surgeons.

- Length of time in the area: A practitioner who has been practicing in the area for a long time is more likely to have good knowledge of other specialists and services in the area that may benefit you.

- Emergency care: Who steps in if he or she is out of town or not available?

Pain Management Clinics

As part of your treatment program, your doctor may refer you to a pain-management clinic. Paula Breuer, a licensed physical therapist at the Centers for Rehabilitation Services, University of Pittsburgh Medical Center, says that many patients think of a pain clinic as a place to get injections and nothing else. "I hear stories from patients who have tried injections, and they didn't help," she said, "so they don't want to be referred to a pain clinic again because they don't want injections."

Although it's true that many pain clinics do give injections, it is also true that many of them are multidisciplinary in nature and are staffed by a range of professionals who offer a combination of both conventional treatments, including medications and injection therapies, and alternative, natural approaches. Some of those techniques, such as acupuncture, biofeedback, chiropractic, guided imagery, hypnosis, hydrotherapy, massage, meditation, and various movement and posture therapies, are discussed in the following chapters.

Before you choose a pain clinic, make sure it is accredited.

Accreditation helps ensure that a clinic's programs meet basic requirements. An accreditation to look for is one assigned by the American Academy of Pain Management, which has a rigorous peer-review process. Pain-management clinics may also be certified by specialty boards such as the American Board of Pain Medicine or the American Board of Anesthesiology.

To find a pain-management clinic in your area, consult your doctor, physical therapist, or hospital. If you have a medical school nearby, check to see if it has a pain clinic. You can also contact the American Pain Society or the American Academy of Pain Medicine (see the resources section).

EVALUATING AND DIAGNOSING CHRONIC LOW BACK PAIN

Many people who have back pain expect two things from their doctors: being told they will need to undergo X-rays and/or other imaging studies and will need medication. Indeed, some people are very disappointed if they don't walk out of their doctor's office with orders for the former and prescriptions for the latter, even though these two approaches to treating chronic low back pain often don't provide adequate pain relief and, in the long run, are costly in terms of both time and money.

I propose that a comprehensive patient history and physical examination, in which the physician asks the right questions, makes careful observations, and performs a hands-on diagnostic evaluation, is the most effective and efficient way to assess a patient's chronic low back pain and thus point the physician toward the most appropriate treatment approach. I further propose that laboratory tests and expensive imaging procedures are vastly overprescribed and, except in specific circumstances, offer little in the way of relevant information. All they often accomplish is a delay in treatment or, at worst, a prescription being written for the wrong kind of treatment, which will overburden already overtaxed health-care and insurance systems.

That being said, let's begin to talk about how I believe chronic low back pain should be diagnosed.

"Red Flag" Signs and Symptoms

Although low back pain can be debilitating and thoroughly disrupt people's lives, it's also true that only about 2 percent of back pain events are medically dangerous and require immediate medical attention. In this small but significant number of cases, the wide spectrum of conditions responsible needs to be identified and ruled out—or ruled in—as the first step of a comprehensive evaluation of a patient's chronic back pain.

Therefore, assessment typically begins by taking a thorough patient history, which includes asking a series of questions whose "yes" answers may indicate the presence of a serious medical condition, such as the following:

- Are you having any trouble controlling bowel function?
- Do you have any newly developed inability to urinate or an increased urgency to urinate?
- Are you experiencing unexplained weakness in your arms, hands, legs, and/or feet?
- Have you lost any sensation in your feet, legs, thighs, groin, or buttocks?
- Do you have new tingling or numbness in your legs or feet?
- Is your back pain constant, never improving somewhat, even when you modify your position?

- Does your back pain wake you up in the middle of the night?
- Do you have a history of cancer?
- Have you recently had a bacterial infection?
- Have you lost weight unintentionally?
- Have you had any unexplained fever or chills?
- Was your back pain previously stable, but you have now experienced sudden and severe worsening of your pain?

A "yes" answer to any of these questions may indicate nerve damage (e.g., cauda equina syndrome), cancer, infection, or an abdominal aortic aneurysm (a weak spot in the aorta, the body's largest artery) and be a sign that your physician needs to investigate the problem further. Remember, serious medical problems as a cause of chronic low back pain are not common, but your physician should explore the possibility, because early diagnosis and treatment of such problems are crucial.

History of Your Back Pain

You can help your health-care professional design an optimal treatment plan if you provide an accurate picture of your back pain history and current state of health. Below are some of the many questions your physician may ask, along with some possible diagnoses. These questions may also reveal conditions that can contribute to or exacerbate your low back pain, such as scoliosis, hip arthritis (which can exacerbate pain associated with the sacroiliac joint), knee arthritis (which can contribute to myofascial pain of the tensor fascia lata), or osteoporosis. These and other conditions, which can be detected during a careful physical examination, are often overlooked in patients who have chronic low back pain, especially older adults. If these conditions are not identified and treated, you could be subjected to unnecessary tests and inappropriate, ineffective treatments.

It is best to review these questions now and think about your answers (you may even want to write them down) so you will be prepared during your visit. While you're sitting in the doctor's office, it can be easy to forget information that your physician may find useful.

The first few questions typically revolve around where the pain is located. These may sound like simple questions, but many patients find that once they really think about their pain, their answers are complicated. As you'll see, your answers can help your doctor narrow down the cause or causes of your back pain.

- Is your pain limited to the lower back? Does it travel to the buttocks and/or down one or both legs? These questions check for sciatica, pain caused by irritation of the sciatic nerve, which runs down the back of the legs. Is the pain sharp or dull? A sharp pain is associated with sciatica, a dull pain with spinal stenosis.
- Do you have pain in your leg(s)? Pain on the sides of the leg, for example, suggests tensor fascia lata/iliotibial band pain if it does not extend beyond the knee, or gluteus minimus myofascial pain if it does. Pain on the sides of the leg accompanied by numbness or tingling indicates that the L5-S1 (fifth lumbar disc, which is the last one before the sacrum) is involved and the source of the radiating pain (radiculopathy). Pain on the front of the thigh suggests hip disease, L2/3/4 radiculopathy (radiating pain source from the second, third, or fourth lumbar disc), or meralgia paresthetica (pinching of the nerve that supplies sensation to the outer thigh).

- Is the pain low (below the waist), over the sacrum to either side of the midline? Pain in the area of the sacrum typically suggests sacroiliac joint syndrome, or much less commonly an inflammatory disorder or a fracture of the sacrum.
- Do you have pain in your buttocks? Such pain may be associated with hip disease, piriformis myofascial pain (in which the piriformis muscle, located deep in the buttocks, is irritated), bursitis, or spinal stenosis.
- Do you have pain in your groin? This pain can be associated with intrinsic hip disease (e.g., arthritis or fracture), myofascial pain, sacroiliac joint syndrome, or a type of common pelvic fracture called an insufficiency fracture of the pubic ramus.
- In addition to low back pain, do you feel pain in many other places in your body? If yes, this may suggest fibromyalgia.

The remaining questions should involve identifying characteristics of your pain.

- How would you rate the pain's severity? You can use a scale of 1 to 10, with 1 being extremely mild and 10 being excruciating. Be sure to tell your physician about changes in severity; for example, the pain may be a 4 when lying down but an 8 when driving or standing. All of these observations are very important in making a diagnosis.
- What makes the pain better? Is the pain better or worse when you lie on your side with your knees curled toward your chest? If there is improvement when you bend forward or are in a curled-up position, for example, it sug-

gests spinal stenosis. If the pain is worse in these positions, it may indicate sacroiliac joint disease. Your answers to these questions may also give clues about whether a nerve is being pressed, possibly related to a herniated disc.

- Is the pain better or worse when you walk? If worse, this suggests spinal stenosis. If it improves the pain, this suggests myofascial pain syndrome or neuropathic (nerve) pain. But these are only indications. Myofascial pain can improve initially when blood circulation to the muscle improves, but it can then get worse if the individual walks too much. Osteoarthritis, especially of the hip, and vascular disease that affects the lower extremities can also worsen with walking. Therefore, your answer to this question can lead a doctor to explore several possibilities.

- When did the pain begin? Was the start of the pain associated with a specific injury or activity? Do you have a history of fracture, back or neck injury, or other trauma, such as an automobile accident or a fall?

- Have you experienced a similar back pain problem in the past? If yes, how was it treated, and was treatment effective?

- Have you ever been diagnosed with other health problems, such as diabetes, hyperthyroidism, fibromyalgia, arthritis, osteoporosis, or cancer? These and other conditions may be associated with low back pain.

Let's Get Physical

I can't emphasize enough the importance of a thorough physical examination. Such an examination should include the following components:

- Visual observation of how you sit, stand, and walk (including how you walk on your toes and on your heels), how you bend forward, sideways, and twist
- Visual evaluation of your posture and curvature of your spine
- Reflex test, in which your doctor uses a little rubber hammer to tap various parts of your lower body to look for clues about possible damage to the spinal cord, nerve roots, or muscles
- Muscle strength test, in which your doctor evaluates the strength of the individual muscle groups of your lower body. Each muscle group is associated with a specific nerve root area of the spine. If a nerve is damaged, then the muscles it controls may indicate some weakness.
- Sensory test, in which your doctor may use a piece of cotton, a pin, or a pinwheel-type device to test symmetrical feeling in your arms and legs. An abnormal response—discomfort, pain, numbness—may indicate a nerve root problem.
- Straight leg test, in which you lie flat on your back with your legs and feet extended on an examining table. The doctor will then slowly lift one of your legs to see if you experience pain in either leg. This test places tension on the sciatic nerve, which runs down the backs of the legs. If you have pain, you may have an irritated nerve root. Some people, however, experience pain because they have tight hamstrings, so the straight leg test is not specific for sciatica-related pain.
- Evaluation for leg length discrepancy
- Hands-on examination (palpation) of the following: sacroiliac joints, myofascial trigger points and fibromyalgia tender points (see figure 2.1), and the piri-

formis muscle, tensor fascia lata and iliotibial band for tightness and pain
- Auscultation (listening with a stethoscope) and palpation of the abdomen, looking for evidence of abdominal aortic aneurysm

Diagnosis: Myofascial Pain Syndrome

One of the main characteristics of myofascial pain, as I discussed in chapter 1, is the presence of trigger points. A diagnosis of myofascial pain implies that specific muscles are responsible for the pain. To make this determination, I palpate (examine with my hands and fingers) certain muscles to see which ones are especially tender. Identifying taut bands and trigger points is helpful because it allows me to tailor an activity or exercise program that will provide optimal pain relief. In fact, people get pain relief when the involved muscle is identified and gently stretched. One pain-relief method called spray and stretch, which involves gentle stretching and the use of a topical medication, is discussed in chapter 7.

There are several types of myofascial trigger points, two of which we will talk about here.

- **Active trigger point** is a site in a muscle or its fascia that is painful and/or tender, whether you are at rest or moving. Such a trigger point prevents you from fully lengthening the affected muscle and is associated with muscle fatigue and decreased strength. When pressure is applied to an active trigger point, it produces and generates the pain (often referred to as stabbing, nagging, aching, or burning in nature), usually in a site *other than the trigger point*. This phenomenon, which is known as *referred* *pain*, is a hallmark of myofascial pain syndrome. In fact, active trigger points are rarely located where the patient reports the pain. The referred pain generated by applying pressure on active trigger points usually has predictable patterns that are specific to each muscle, which helps in diagnosis. You might think of referred pain as the dynamite that explodes when someone at a remote site pushes the detonator button (in this case, the trigger point).

- **Latent trigger point** is one that does not cause pain during normal activities but does when palpated. It also refers pain when pressure is applied. It is believed that latent trigger points are common in the general population. A latent trigger point can develop into an active one for several reasons, including the presence of muscle tension, psychological stress, and poor posture, all of which can contribute to or cause low back pain.

The identification of trigger points and the resulting referred pain patterns are a joint effort between the physician and the patient. My job is to use my sense of touch (palpation) to locate highly sensitive nodules of muscle fiber and to observe the patient's response to the pain, which is usually an involuntary withdrawal (called a jump sign) when I apply pressure. This is a strong indication that I have located a trigger point. If I continue to apply pressure on the trigger point for several seconds or as long as a minute, the patient usually experiences the same referred pain that brought him or her to my office. Another sign of a trigger point is a local twitch response—a rapid contraction of the muscle fibers of the taut band that contains a trigger point. The role of the patient is to report on the level of pain associated with the palpation of each point and the referred pain that results. Once the trigger points and pain patterns have been identified, treatment options can be discussed. Effective treatments for myofascial pain syndrome include digital pressure, acupuncture, spray and stretch, trigger-point injection, application of heat and/or cold, and a variety of other therapies covered in chapters 3 through 5.

Diagnosis: Fibromyalgia

A diagnosis of fibromyalgia is based on a history of widespread pain that persists for more than three months and is accompanied by tenderness in at least eleven of eighteen specific tender points on the body (see figure 2.1), one of the criteria established by the American College of Rheumatology to classify fibromyalgia. The notion of needing eleven of eighteen tender points was developed to differentiate fibromyalgia from other rheumatologic disorders that are also characterized by widespread pain, such as systemic lupus erythematosus and rheumatoid arthritis, and not to diagnose fibromyalgia per se. Therefore, I don't believe this criterion should be the one to make or break a patient's diagnosis. It is more important, in my opinion, to look for commonly associated symptoms and the patient's overall condition. Seventy-five percent of patients have fatigue, morning stiffness, and nonrestorative sleep. If patients come to me with these symptoms along with generalized pain, but do not have at least eleven tender points, I treat them for fibromyalgia anyway.

To determine whether a patient has tender points, I palpate each of the identified points, which can be seen in the accompanying figure. Patients often describe the pain as throbbing, shooting, stabbing, or aching, sometimes with a feeling of severe burning. Typically, the pain and stiffness are more pronounced in the morning.

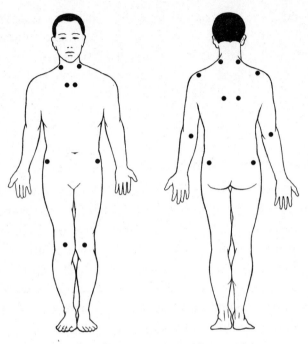

Figure 2.1 Tender points of fibromyalgia

Pain and tenderness are not the only characteristic indications of fibromyalgia, however. Other signs and symptoms, and how they compare with those associated with myofascial pain syndrome, are listed in the table below. In fact, myofascial pain is common in patients who have fibromyalgia, and indeed fibromyalgia syndrome and myofascial pain syndrome frequently occur together.

Some individuals report the symptoms of fibromyalgia beginning shortly after they have been in an automobile accident or experienced similar physical trauma, while others say symptoms began after they recovered from an infection, such as the flu or a urinary tract infection. Yet other cases seem to appear along with the development of another disorder, such as lupus, chronic fatigue syndrome, hypothyroidism, or rheumatoid arthritis. It's unclear whether such events cause fibromyalgia or simply trigger an existing, underlying abnormality experts have not yet identified.

Differences Between Myofascial Pain Syndrome and Fibromyalgia

Feature	Myofascial	Fibromyalgia
Trigger/tender points	Localized	Generalized
Trigger points	Have nodular feel	
Tender points		No specific characteristics
Pain	Localized	Generalized
Referred pain	Very common	Less common
Fatigue	Less common	Very common
Poor sleep	Less common; due to pain	Very common; due to neuroendocrine imbalance
Headache	Less common	Very common
Irritable bowel	Less common	Very common
Brain "fog"	Much less common	Very common

Diagnosis: Lumbar Spinal Stenosis

As I mentioned in chapter 1, spinal stenosis is a narrowing of the spinal canal, which causes nerves that run to the legs and buttocks to be "pinched." Indications that you may have lumbar spinal stenosis are the following:

- Your back and leg/buttocks pain goes away or is greatly relieved when you lean forward at the waist when you walk. One indication is leaning on the shopping cart in the grocery store because it makes your back feel better.

- You find it difficult to walk quickly and/or to walk any great distance.
- You get relief if you sit down.

Diagnosis: Degenerated Discs or Facet Joints

Degeneration of vertebral discs and/or facet joints can appear in people of any age, although it is more common among individuals older than forty. Indications that you may have one or more degenerated vertebral discs or facet joints include the following:

- Pain that increases when you bend, sit, or lift
- Presence of low back pain and stiffness
- Pain that may radiate down the legs and into the feet and be associated with numbness and tingling

Diagnosis: Herniated Disc

The good news about this common back problem is that it heals well with proper therapy and time. Indications that you may have a herniated (bulging, ruptured) disc include the following:

- Sharp, cutting pain that gets worse as it moves down the leg
- Pain that increases when you cough, sneeze, ride in a car, or flex your trunk
- Limited range of motion when you bend forward or backward
- Pain that came on suddenly
- Pain, weakness, and/or numbness in one or both legs

Diagnosis: Vertebral Compression Fracture

A compression fracture is one cause of chronic back pain that is most often seen in older adults. Indications that you may have a compression fracture include the following:

- Pain that increases with activity. This is not always a good indication, but it should be considered.
- Pain that wakes you up at night
- Weakness, tingling, or numbness in one or both legs
- Pain that does not decrease a week or two after it first appeared
- Pain that occurred suddenly or immediately after bending or lifting, or following minor trauma or a fall. This is especially true in older individuals.

Hip Arthritis and Back Pain

When a patient complains of back pain, and especially when that patient is around sixty-five or older, osteoarthritis of the hip is frequently a cause. Yet many physicians miss a diagnosis of hip arthritis and instead treat patients, unsuccessfully, for low back pain. You can help your physician differentiate your back pain from hip arthritis by explaining your pain as clearly as possible and noting any other symptoms. Indications I check for and ask patients about include gait problems, clicking in the hip, a hip that "gives way," muscle weakness, and pain in the buttocks, groin, thigh, or knee. Generally, hip arthritis also causes limited and painful hip motion. Patients complain that their hip is stiff, especially after inactivity, which makes it difficult to perform certain tasks, such as putting on shoes and socks.

DIAGNOSTIC TESTS

My stance, as you might have guessed by now, is that laboratory tests and imaging procedures should be used judiciously. Much too often, patients are subjected to costly and unnecessary testing, a situation that is upsetting to me and also is significant because it not only wastes precious health-care resources, it also dupes people into believing they have been given an answer to their pain. The penchant for testing has lead to a failure among many physicians to recognize some conditions, because they focus on technology rather than taking the time for tried-and-true, solid basics: touching, talking with, and understanding their patients.

That being said, there is a place for diagnostic tests to help rule out serious medical conditions as the cause of chronic back pain. Indeed, as I explained in chapter 1, in a small minority of patients, the presence of an infection; malignancy; more unusual rheumatologic diseases, such as ankylosing spondylitis or psoriatic arthritis; or a neurologic disorder can be identified as the cause of chronic back pain. We also need to keep in mind, however, that these test results can sometimes be misleading. Thus, it takes a knowledgeable practitioner to carefully weigh a patient's history and the information gathered from the physical examination and personal consultation against any test results, if indeed the physician has decided tests are necessary.

Body Chemistry Testing

The tests in this category should be used when a physician suspects that an infection or a malignancy is the cause of back pain.

- **Blood tests:** Various blood tests, including a complete blood count (CBC), erythrocyte sedimentation rate (ESR), and others are used to screen for serious diseases that can cause or contribute to back pain.
- **Urinalysis:** An abnormal finding on a urinalysis can suggest many different urinary problems that are associated with back pain, including kidney stones, infections, blockages, and tumors.

To Image or Not to Image

The truth is that many people who are without back pain have the same abnormal findings on their X-rays and MRI scans as do people who have chronic low back pain. This fact should make health professionals and consumers stop and think about the diagnostic value of MRIs. In one study, for example, MRI scans showed herniated discs in about 25 percent of people younger than sixty who had no back pain symptoms and in 33 percent of pain-free people older than sixty. In a prospective study published in 2001, investigators at the University of Washington, Seattle, assessed the MRI scans of 148 randomly selected outpatients. Sixty-nine (46 percent) had never experienced low back pain, yet 123 showed moderate to severe damage to one or more discs, 95 (64 percent) had one or more bulging discs, and 48 (32 percent) had at least one disc protrusion. The researchers concluded that MRI findings are of limited diagnostic value in low back pain.

It's also true that imaging techniques such as X-rays and MRIs cannot provide a definitive diagnosis for back pain that is muscle-related, which makes up a significant proportion of cases. Overall, therefore, I suggest MRIs be used to look for infections or cancer or in patients who require surgery, while plain X-rays, not MRIs, should be used to diagnose skeletal problems, such as compression fractures.

Every year, seven to eight million lumbosacral spine imaging series are ordered in the United States. Unfortunately, most of these tests offer physicians very little information that can help them decide on a course of treatment for their patients, especially among people younger than fifty, who make up the majority of individuals who have chronic low back pain. In addition, these tests expose individuals to excessive radiation, three thousand units more than occurs during a chest X-ray. Yet another concern is that these tests are very expensive and place an undue burden on an already overextended health-care system.

Imaging and Nerve Conduction Techniques

Here's an introduction to the more common imaging and nerve-testing techniques used in the diagnosis of chronic back pain.

X-rays. Conventional X-rays, or radiographs, are used primarily to show abnormalities of bone, such as fractures, arthritis, and slippage. To capture such an image, a beam of energy is aimed at the designated body site, and a plate that has been placed behind the body part captures the variations of the beam as it passes through internal structures. X-rays cannot show soft tissues, such as muscles, intervertebral discs, and ligaments. Therefore, X-rays are not useful in diagnosing the majority of back pain situations. If infection, a tumor, or nerve compression is suspected, it is best to have an MRI and not an X-ray, as these conditions cannot be seen on X-rays. X-rays may be indicated, however, if any of the following are true for you:

- Medical history of cancer, alcohol or drug abuse, or corticosteroid use
- Unusual/unexplained weight loss
- Fever
- History of serious physical trauma
- Evidence of nerve problems your doctor observed during the neurologic examination
- Suspicion of ankylosing spondylitis, a type of arthritis in which the vertebrae gradually fuse together until the spine is rigid. It is also sometimes called frozen spine or poker spine.
- Sudden worsening of stable pain

Computed Tomography. A CT scan is a diagnostic tool that uses computer-enhanced radiation to produce images that are clearer and more detailed than those produced during regular X-rays. That's because the X-ray beam of a CT scan moves around the body part, taking many different views of the same area and providing an image with much more detail. The images are processed by a computer and displayed on a monitor.

CT scans are often ordered when a physician suspects disc rupture, vertebra damage, or spinal stenosis. These scans can be taken with or without contrast media. Use of contrast—a substance taken orally or injected into an intravenous line prior to the procedure—allows the site under study to be seen more clearly. Although CT scans produce better images of soft tissues than do regular X-rays, they are not as sophisticated as MRI scans, which we discuss below. They are like MRIs, however, in that they often show back abnormalities in people who are pain-free.

Magnetic Resonance Imaging. A nonradiation approach to imaging is magnetic resonance imaging, which, unlike X-rays and CT, uses radio waves in a magnetic field to produce images. An MRI can provide very clear images of intervertebral discs, tumors, infections, and damage to the spinal cord. However, many people have abnormalities in their back that either do not cause pain or are not the cause of the pain they are experiencing. Many patients feel "cheated" if their doctor doesn't order an MRI when they complain of back pain. It's important for people to know that MRIs often are not necessary and that even if an MRI were to show an abnormality, very often that abnormality would not correlate with their symptoms. A study published in the *New England Journal of Medicine* illustrates this. Of ninety-eight pain-free individuals who had a lumbar spine MRI, only 36 percent had normal discs. Therefore, 64 percent of the MRIs showed abnormalities that could be associated with back pain, yet none of the individuals had such pain.

Myelography. This technique involves the injection of a contrast medium into the fluid-filled sac around the spinal cord, after which X-rays are taken. If the X-rays identify any reduction or blockage of the flow of the cerebrospinal fluid in your spinal column, it indicates that there is pressure on the nerves of the spine, possibly from a bony spur, a herniated disc, or a tumor. This test can be especially helpful in diagnosing lumbar spinal stenosis. A myelogram takes about one hour to complete. Your doctor may also order a CT scan as part of your myelogram (a CT-myelogram), which can provide additional information that a myelogram alone may not show.

The main drawback of having a myelogram is the risk of getting a spinal headache, which is caused by a change in the pressure of the cerebrospinal fluid. If a spinal headache does occur, it can be treated with rest and plenty of fluids and usually lasts one or two days.

Electromyelography (EMG). This test studies the condition of the nerve roots leaving the spine by examining the electrical activity in the muscles these nerves control. With lower back pain, your doctor may test your leg muscles to see if there is a problem with the nerves that send signals to your legs. An EMG involves placing tiny needles into various muscles to evaluate their electrical activity. If the electrical activity in the muscle is abnormal, it may indicate that a nerve is being pinched or irritated, which in turn suggests spinal stenosis or a herniated disc.

An EMG takes from thirty to sixty minutes to complete, depending on the number of muscles tested. Although there are no major risks involved in undergoing this test, it does cause some discomfort, and I believe it is not very reliable when it comes to identifying which nerve is compressed. An EMG is often ordered along with a nerve-conduction study, discussed below.

Bone Scan. This imaging technique is used to diagnose and monitor infections, fractures, and bone disorders. Before a scan is done, a small amount of radioactive substance is injected into the bloodstream. This substance collects in the bones, which are then scanned to identify specific areas of abnormal bone metabolism, unusual blood flow, or joint disease.

I believe bone scans are generally unnecessary unless a patient experiences an acute episode of chronic pain that is unusually severe or that wakes him or her from sleep. In such cases, I would order regular X-rays, and if the X-rays didn't reveal a problem, I would seriously consider a bone scan. While it is not uncommon for people to experience acute flares of chronic pain, a flare that is more severe than individuals typically experience suggests something more serious may be happening.

Nerve-Conduction Study. This study, which I believe is greatly overused, is often ordered as part of a comprehensive nerve and muscle diagnostic test. A nerve-conduction study involves placing two sets of small electrodes on the skin over the muscles to be tested. The first set of electrodes sends a mild shock to stimulate the nerve that runs to a specific muscle. The second set of electrodes records the nerve's electrical signals, which are evaluated to determine whether there is nerve damage and to measure the extent of the damage. The electrical signals are picked up by a computer, and the information is interpreted by a physician, who should have your results within a few days.

LOST IN TRANSLATION: TALKING BACK

As if diagnosing back pain wasn't complicated enough, you may find that physicians and other health-care practitioners often use different terms to talk about the same condition. For example, one practitioner may look at your MRI and say you have a herniated disc, while another practitioner may call it a bulging disc, slipped disc, or prolapsed disc. Physicians often use these terms interchangeably, and this practice can be very confusing for patients and even other practitioners.

Adding to the confusion of back talk is the use of misleading terminology for different conditions. For example, degenerative disc disease is not a disease but a condition that can, but may not, produce pain. While everyone can expect their discs to deteriorate to varying degrees as they age, it is by no means a given that everyone will develop painful symptoms associated with deterioration. Another confusing phrase is failed back surgery syndrome, which is not a syndrome at all, but a condition in which a patient still has pain even though he or she has undergone a procedure that was meant to significantly reduce or eliminate the pain (see chapter 8).

One "cure" for translation difficulties is to ask questions: If you don't understand what your doctor is telling you, ask him or her to describe it again. If your doctor uses terms that confuse you, ask for clarification; if he mentions specific muscles, for example, ask him to show you where they are so you can associate the names with a visual memory. Another cure is to do your homework: read books, articles, and information from reputable Web sites and organizations about back pain. (Some suggestions can be found in the resources section.) You have a right to accurate information about your own health.

DIAGNOSING DEPRESSION

One of the first things I learned during my early days as a physician was that many people who have chronic pain experience significant pain relief and improved quality of life when they are treated with antidepressants. This is true not only because antidepressants can relieve pain, but also because *many people suffer with undiagnosed—and therefore untreated—depression, and untreated depression in individuals with chronic pain exacerbates their pain and contributes to a deterioration in their quality of life*. Thus, I believe it is vitally important for physicians to evaluate patients who are living with chronic back pain for signs and symptoms of depression and anxiety and, if present, to immediately treat them for these conditions. (See the box Signs and Symptoms of Depression.) Failure to do so can jeopardize any therapy and treatment efforts to relieve and prevent further back pain. In fact, it's important for people to understand that treating the pain alone is not enough. Many people think they are depressed because they are in pain, and if the pain is significantly reduced, their depression will improve as well. Unfortunately, this often is not the case, which is why I encourage a more proactive approach to the treatment of depression in patients who have chronic low back pain.

Signs and Symptoms of Depression

The accepted criteria for major depression, as defined in the *Diagnostic and Statistical Manual of Mental Disorders*, Fourth Edition (DSM-IV), is that at least five of the following symptoms occur daily for at least two weeks. The symptoms include:

- A predominant mood characterized by sadness, feeling blue or hopeless, irritability, feeling low or depressed
- Significant change in appetite and/or weight; either poor appetite and significant weight loss or increased appetite and weight gain
- Sleep problems—too much sleep or too little sleep
- Loss of interest in activities that once brought pleasure
- Decreased or loss of interest in sex
- Feeling fatigued or restless
- Feeling guilty and/or worthless
- Memory or concentration difficulties
- Thoughts of suicide, death, or wishing to be dead

People with chronic pain are three to four times as likely to have depression or anxiety as people who are pain-free. One study showed that an average of 62 percent of patients with chronic low back pain who sought help at a pain clinic were depressed. A 2004 study found that the rate of major depression increased as pain severity increased. Yet the reality is that primary care physicians and other practitioners who are diagnosing and treating back pain often miss the indicators of clinical depression and suicidal thoughts. At the same time, people with chronic back pain who are depressed often are not aware they are depressed.

This was certainly the case with Lillian, a sixty-eight-year-old widow who had retired three years earlier from her job as an automobile manufacturing manager in Pittsburgh, where she had spent decades walking on concrete floors and suffering with low back pain. Her long-awaited retirement was marred by chronic pain that prevented her from even simple pleasures, such as playing with her grandchildren. She had been diagnosed with lumbar spinal stenosis when she was fifty-five, and over the years had undergone several series of epidural steroid injections, which had provided some relief each time that had then faded.

When Lillian came to see me, she was brought in by her daughter-in-law, Carla, who said her mother-in-law was growing increasingly depressed and that her pain was not under control. At that time, Lillian was taking the NSAID naproxen along with acetaminophen and was not participating in any type of physical therapy program. "My mother-in-law is terrified to do any type of exercise," said Carla. "She's convinced she will only hurt more. She's missing out on enjoying her grandchildren, and she won't go out to see her friends."

Lillian's depression and fear of activity were contributing to her pain and disability, so we needed to boost her mood while easing her back into physical activity. I started her on an antidepressant (citalopram, or Celexa) and referred her to a psychologist for cognitive-behavioral therapy to help her learn coping skills and to get over her fear. At first, Lillian resisted going to the psychologist because, she said, "I'm not crazy, I just hurt." Only after a friend of hers admitted to going to a therapist did Lillian consent to the sessions. After two weeks, I added physical therapy to the program, which included massage and stretching exercises. Within six weeks, Carla said her mother-in-law was a different person.

"Her mood is 100 percent better," said Carla. "She's doing her exercises, and she says her pain is about 50 percent better. This is a great improvement. She's even talking about taking a trip to California to see her sister."

Double Trouble

It's not hard to see how having chronic back pain can send individuals down the spiral road to major depression. Consider this:

- The pain interferes with sleep, which makes you overly tired and cranky.
- The pain makes it difficult to participate in activities you once enjoyed or needed to participate in. This inability adds to your sense of frustration.
- You may find you are more and more isolated from others, including family, friends, and co-workers, because you don't feel well enough or are unable to participate in family and social events.

- You may be unable to work or find it difficult to work, which may be placing you in a negative financial situation.
- The pain may make it difficult for you to concentrate.
- Medications you may be taking for the pain may be causing adverse effects, such as gastrointestinal distress, drowsiness, memory problems, vision problems, and sleep difficulties.
- Your desire for or ability to participate in sexual activities may have disappeared, which can place a great deal of stress on your personal relationship.

If you recognize signs of depression in your life, talk to your doctor. Treatment with the right antidepressant could reduce your back pain, lift your mood, and improve your overall quality of life.

DEMENTIA AND BACK PAIN

As the population of older adults continues to increase, so does the number of people who have dementia. It takes a specially trained eye to properly evaluate and treat these individuals when it comes to concomitant conditions, such as chronic low back pain. Family members and caregivers can be very helpful to physicians who face the challenge of diagnosing and treating patients who have dementia and who are unable to verbally communicate information about their pain. Thus, if you have a loved one who has dementia and you suspect he or she has back pain, your input can make a significant difference. Input from caregivers at a nursing facility can also be critical.

For example, you can make sure the physician has a complete medical history of your loved one, including past surgeries and medication use. You can consult with the physician about any potential causes of pain that may not appear in the history, such as an automobile accident or a fall. You may also know about behaviors the patient has shown in the past when he or she was in pain. Another important source of information is the nursing home staff who are caring for your loved one. A study conducted at the Research Institute on Aging in Rockville, Maryland, found that caregiving staff who are familiar with a resident can provide critical information for physicians who are trying to identify pain behavior.

Researchers have also developed some guidelines to help health-care professionals identify when nonverbal patients with dementia are in pain. At the University of Wisconsin–Milwaukee, researchers have created the Assessment of Discomfort in Dementia (ADD) plan, which is put into action when an individual displays certain behaviors that suggest he or she is in pain, including increased agitation, fidgeting, or repetitive movements; tense muscles and/or bracing the body; increased or repetitive verbalizations; decreased cognition; changes in sleep habits; increase in heart rate, blood pressure, and sweating; and decreased functional ability or withdrawal. If any of these behaviors are apparent, physicians are prompted to do the following:

1. Look for physical causes for discomfort, such as infection, inflammation, and chronic conditions.
2. Review the patient's history, and consult with family members and/or caregivers about any additional information that may help with the evaluation.
3. If no physical reasons can be found for discomfort, use nondrug interventions, such as physical exercise, soothing touch, music therapy, and therapeutic massage.

These measures can reduce the patient's stress, which may be contributing to or be the sole source of discomfort.

4. If the nondrug interventions are not successful in relieving the individual's discomfort, try non-narcotic painkillers, such as acetaminophen.

5. If this effort does not bring about a positive response, consider that a stronger painkiller or a psychotropic drug may be needed.

IN CONCLUSION . . .

I firmly believe that the vast majority of individuals who have chronic low back pain can be diagnosed accurately without resorting to many of the imaging and other testing procedures so often prescribed today. Rather, careful observation; a thorough, comprehensive physical examination; and evaluation of your history and lifestyle by a knowledgeable health-care practitioner can best identify the one or more factors associated with your chronic pain. Your physician can then quickly put you on a healing path, whereas a superficial assessment and unnecessary testing can prevent you from getting the pain relief you need and deserve and can prove costly as well.

That being said, we now turn to a detailed discussion of a six-step treatment program that includes the options for chronic low back pain that I have found to be effective.

Part II

SIX STEPS TO
BACK PAIN RELIEF

In the next several chapters, I describe my six-step approach to the management of chronic back pain. If there's only one message readers get from this section, it should be that a multidisciplinary approach—which may or may not include the use of medications—can be very effective in the treatment of chronic low back pain. My six-step approach to the treatment of chronic back pain begins with and focuses on noninvasive, nonpharmacological methods, methods I believe should be the first line of attack against back pain in nearly every case. Once a diagnosis has been made, I encourage patients to work with health-care professionals as they select and try various modalities, beginning with a basic home exercise program, and then adding on other options, from hydrotherapy to acupuncture, Pilates, TENS, yoga, biofeedback, and meditation—even injection therapies and medications as needed to further advance the rehabilitation process.

One interesting thing about the many different noninvasive, nondrug options is that, like their counterparts, what works for some people may not work for others. Some of my patients swear by acupuncture or yoga, while others say, "They didn't work for me, but let me tell you how wonderful Feldenkrais makes me feel" or "Meditation and an exercise program have been the answer for me." It's clearly a matter of different strokes for different folks. Some patients find they need to take medication temporarily when they first start physical therapy; others do well without it. Every case is unique, and every individual has different needs, expectations, and goals. My purpose in these chapters is to introduce the possibilities to you (illustrated throughout with stories from patients who have used these techniques), encourage you to try those that interest you or that meet your needs, and hope you will find relief from chronic back pain, as so many of my patients have.

I also want to make it clear that, if you find you need injections and/or medications, they should be viewed not as an end in and of themselves but as a way to facilitate your exercise program and rehabilitation, which lead to improved function and a better quality of life. Another important point is that use of medications should *always* be combined with nonpharmacological approaches, which can not only enhance the efficacy of any drugs you are taking but also reduce the dosage, frequency, and/or number of drugs you need to take. Reducing the need for medications while maintaining adequate pain control is of major importance, given that use of multiple medications and any side effects from these drugs can have an extremely detrimental impact on quality of life. Indeed, it is not unusual for adverse reactions to drugs to prevent patients from being able to participate in an exercise program or physical therapy or to cause them to lose motivation to continue with such activities, even when they are physically able to do so.

Chapter 3

Step 1: Let's Get Physical

In my experience, a well-orchestrated plan of exercise and physical therapy can be the best medicine for people who have chronic low back pain. Yet very often, these approaches are given cursory attention by both physicians and patients, who are not offered an opportunity to benefit from such a plan. Many patients shy away from exercise and physical therapy because they are afraid the movement and activity will hurt too much or, worse yet, cause them harm and result in further disability. In fact, the opposite is the case, especially when patients work with a physical therapist to develop an activity plan that addresses their specific needs and condition.

Although the days when doctors ordered weeks of bed rest for back pain are thankfully pretty much in the past, a proactive program of physical therapy and exercise has not replaced it in many cases. Yet even the most reluctant patients, once they incorporate exercise and other physical activities into their lives, often cannot stop telling others how much better they feel and how exercise has been "the answer" to improving their quality of life and reducing their pain.

In this chapter, I attempt to awaken an appreciation for the benefits physical therapy and exercise have to offer you and others who suffer with chronic back pain. Our discussion of physical therapy looks at three categories. First, we look at the most important category—movement therapy, or the "E" word, exercise. The good news is that simple works: you don't need fancy equipment or an expensive health club membership to take excellent care of your back when it comes to exercise. I'll show you some stretching and strengthening exercises, including instructions and illustrations for selected movements where appropriate, and several movement therapies. You should, of course, consult your doctor or physical therapist before starting any exercise or movement program.

Next, we look at what can be called "assisted therapies," which include ultrasound, hydrotherapy, application of heat and cold, traction, spinal manipulation, and TENS. These therapies are often applied or facilitated by a therapist, but patients can certainly perform them alone as well. Besides being effective in relieving pain and associated symptoms of back pain, these passive therapies are often used to complement a home exercise program.

The third category is physical devices worn on the body as a means of support and stabilization and includes braces, belts, corsets, and orthotics. I explain the conditions each can benefit and the advantages and drawbacks of use.

GETTING PHYSICAL

In recent years, doctors and other medical professionals have recognized the value of exercise in the prevention and treatment of low back pain. Quite simply, it works when approached responsibly and under the guidance of a knowledgeable professional. Once experts have diagnosed your back problem and developed an exercise program that fulfills your specific needs, limitations, and physical condition, it's up to you to do the work, with their assistance and advice, as needed.

Getting Motivated

Scores of studies support this view of the role of exercise in back pain, and various exercise programs and methods are available to help people meet it, several of which we discuss in this chapter. The challenge I often face in my practice, as do my colleagues, is in *motivating patients to exercise.* I understand their reluctance: people who live with chronic pain are not especially motivated to do things they believe will cause them more pain. I agree. *Exercise should not hurt, and it doesn't have to.* But I know that if they do exercise, they may be working toward hurting less or, even if their pain doesn't subside significantly, exercise can help them function better, build strength and endurance, improve flexibility, and improve their quality of life overall.

A physical therapist can help you with both the exercise program and complementary treatments to make your exercise sessions more comfortable and effective and help keep you motivated in the process. Paula Breuer, L.P.T., a physical therapist at the Centers for Rehabilitation Services at the University of Pittsburgh Medical Center, explains that many people don't understand that the pain they may feel when they begin to exercise or go to physical therapy is not a sign of injury, but a sign of not having used their muscles or perhaps exercising or stretching a little too intensely. "Most people stop exercising when they feel the pain," she says. "At that point, they are irritating their tissues, and if they continue the exercise, they will have more irritation."

This is the time when motivation can be a problem, and many people turn to medication—painkillers, muscle relaxants, anti-inflammatory drugs—either over-the-counter or prescriptions from their doctor. Guidance and explanations by a physical therapist about what your muscles and body are going through during physical therapy can be comforting and reassuring. Paula Breuer and I agree that drugs usually are not the answer. "People don't always need pain medication to get through their exercises," she says, "but rather a modification of the exercises. This means patients need to work very closely with their physical therapist to make those changes." Along with modification of your exercise program, and even before you begin a program, your physical therapist can treat you with various other therapies, such as massage, hydrotherapy, ultrasound, and the application of cold/heat, that can reduce your pain and help make your exercise sessions more enjoyable and productive. We discuss these and other techniques later in this chapter under Physical Therapy.

I strongly encourage patients to utilize and take advantage of the services of a physical therapist. If your doctor prescribes therapy, go. If he or she does not, ask about it. The ideal situation is one-on-one sessions with a therapist, although this may not be feasible because of cost or insurance restrictions, or the facility may not have sufficient staff to devote much individual attention to patients. However, try to find a clinic or practice in which the physical therapist works with you as closely as possible and educates you about each exercise as you learn and perform it. This type of attention not only helps you heal faster and more efficiently but encourages you to stay with your exercise program.

Benefits of Exercise

In addition to building strength, endurance, range of motion, and flexibility related to the back muscles and associated structures, daily exercise stimulates production of the body's natural painkillers, called endorphins. It also reduces emotional and mental stress, improves mood, and if weight is a problem, helps drop pounds. To reap the benefits of exercise when you live with chronic low back pain, you need a combination of movements that are right for your specific condition. That combination should be determined by your physician and physical therapist. However, we can look at some of the many options available to you so you can discuss them with health-care professionals and even try some exercises on your own (with your doctor's permission, of course).

Let's Do It!

I believe exercise should be as safe and fun as possible. For safety, consult with your doctor and/or physical therapist about which exercises and activities are best for your condition and abilities. With that thought in mind, your approach to an exercise program is best done in two steps. One is the development stage, during which you work with a physical therapist to identify your strengths and weaknesses and put together an exercise program that contains the types of exercises that will best suit your needs, information on how to do them correctly, and any complementary therapies that may help with this process. Paula Breuer notes that one of the reasons exercise programs fail is because people want to rush: they try to exercise at the level they did *before* their present condition. In the program she facilitates, patients begin with a few stretches and some walking and do not begin aerobic and strength exercises until the end of week three of their six-week program. Thus, the emphasis is on working slowly and pacing properly to get the maximum benefit.

The second step is the maintenance program, which is the plan you will follow once the development stage is complete. Generally, a well-rounded maintenance exercise program includes a five- to ten-minute warm-up (e.g., light stretching or slow walking on a treadmill), followed by twenty to thirty minutes of an aerobic activity, such as brisk walking, rowing, swimming, dancing, biking, or jogging, and is capped off with five minutes of light stretching again. You may want to vary your aerobic activity to help keep it interesting. Some patients find it difficult to get out of the house to exercise and opt to follow along with an aerobic video at home. This can be a great option if you check with your health-care professional to make sure the movements will not harm you.

Every other day, the aerobic session should be replaced by strengthening exercises that may or may not involve the use of light weights and/or equipment. If you use weights or equipment, an expert who is knowledgeable about back conditions should help you use them properly, as weights and exercise equipment can place a great deal of stress on the lower back and cause harm if they are used incorrectly.

The intensity and choice of exercises and physical activities that you and your health-care professional choose will be tailored to your needs. As you participate in your program, you may need to make adjustments, depending on how you feel and the progress you make. It's important, however, that you make these exercises a regular part of your lifestyle so you can help maintain a healthy, strong back.

Some of the more common strengthening and stretching exercises are described here and illustrated on pages 85–90. *Please consult your health-care professional before you do any of these exercises.* The floor exercises are best done using an exercise mat or, if you don't have a mat, on top of several layers of blankets or large towels. (Patients who have difficulty getting down and up from the floor can use a bed or couch to do the floor exercises.) The number of repetitions given here are suggestions only. Your health-care professional will determine the best program for you. (Remember: Always stretch first!)

- **The Cat** (figure 3.1; stretches and loosens muscles, strengthens back and abdominal muscles): Get down on the floor on all fours, with your back flat and your weight distributed evenly. Your neck should be parallel to the floor. Inhale through your nose as you arch your back upward by tightening your abdominal and buttocks muscles. Your head will drop slightly. Hold this position for a count of five. Then exhale through your mouth as you let your back relax and sag gently toward the floor. Hold this position for a count of five. Repeat the entire sequence up to five times. Remember to keep your arms straight and your weight evenly distributed throughout the exercise. (Note: Talk to your physical therapist before doing this exercise if you have knee problems.)
- **Knee Cross** (figure 3.2; stretches the lower back and hips): Lie on your left side and extend both legs. You can

place your right hand on the floor in front of you to help support your body. Bend your right (top) knee and pull it toward your chest so that your right foot is near your left knee. Press your right knee across your left leg and down toward the floor. Then raise your right knee toward the ceiling until you feel a stretch. Keep your right foot on your left knee and hold for at least five seconds. Then lower your top knee and return to the starting position. Repeat the entire exercise from the beginning three to five times, then turn onto your right side and repeat all the steps with your left leg.

- **Wall Slide** (figure 3.3; strengthens back, calf, and thigh muscles): Stand with your back against a wall, with your feet shoulder-width apart and one foot away from the wall. Tighten your buttocks muscles and press your lower back into the wall. Place your hands on your hips. Slowly bend your knees and slide your back down the wall partway toward a seated position. Only go down as far as you can without causing pain. If you experience pain, slide down a little less the next time. Hold the position for five seconds, then slowly slide back up the wall. (Note: If you need some help when sliding down the wall, press your arms against the wall behind you and keep your palms flat.)

- **Leg Raises, Face Down** (figure 3.4; strengthens lower back and back of the thighs): Lie on your stomach on a firm, padded surface with your legs straight and together and your arms at your sides. Contract your buttocks muscles and lift your right leg off the mat as high as you can without bending your knee. (Do not allow your pelvic bones to rise off the mat while you lift your leg.) Hold your leg in the raised position for five seconds, then lower it to the mat. Repeat with the left leg. Do five repetitions with each leg. (Note: This exercise should not be done if you have spinal stenosis and can be very difficult if you have kyphosis or limited extension in your legs. Talk to your physical therapist before doing this exercise. He or she may recommend placing a pillow under your pelvis when doing this exercise.)

- **Mini Sit-Up** (figure 3.5; strengthens the stomach muscles): Lie on your back on a firm, padded surface with your knees bent and your arms at your sides. Contract your stomach muscles and raise your head, neck, and shoulders off the floor. Stretch your arms out straight and reach with your hands to your knees. Keep your eyes on the ceiling and don't bend your neck. When your shoulders are off the floor, hold that position for two or three seconds, then return your shoulders, neck, and head to the floor. Repeat ten times. (Note: If you have osteoporosis, talk to your physical therapist before doing this exercise.)

- **Pelvic Lift** (figure 3.6; strengthens the buttocks and abdominal muscles; stabilizes the trunk): Lie on your back with your knees bent and your feet about eighteen inches apart. Your soles should be flat on the floor and your arms should be by your sides. Contract your buttocks muscles and slowly lift your pelvis off the floor until your spine forms a straight line from your neck to your knees. Do not arch your back. Hold that position for five seconds; then, beginning with your shoulder area, slowly lower your back, allowing one vertebra at a time to touch the floor until your tailbone is the last one to touch. Repeat this exercise five times.

- **Leg Raises** (figure 3.7; strengthens the stomach muscles and stretches the lower back and back of the thighs): Lie flat on your back with your arms at your sides. Bend your left knee and keep your right leg straight. Raise your right leg as high as you can without lifting your hips off the floor and without increasing pain. Hold your right leg at the highest position for five seconds, then slowly lower it to the floor. Repeat the leg raise with the right leg five more times, then bend the right knee, straighten the left leg, and do the raises with the left leg.

- **Roll Back** (figure 3.8; helps relieve stress in the back): Lie on your back with your knees bent and your feet flat on the floor. Your head should remain on the floor throughout this exercise. Lift your knees, place both hands under them, and gently pull your knees toward your chest as close as possible. Hold this position for a second or two, then lower one leg to the floor, then the other, while keeping your knees bent, returning to your starting position. Repeat the exercise five times, several times a day, to help relieve tension in your back.

Water Aerobics

The next prescription you get from your doctor could read as follows: "Put on a bathing suit and walk, jog, or Jazzercise in a warm pool for thirty to forty minutes three times a week." Water aerobics, a form of hydrotherapy, is one of the best exercise treatments for people who have chronic low back pain, because the buoyancy of the water supports much of the body's weight and thus takes stress off the joints. If you are in chest-deep water, 75 percent of your body weight is supported; at

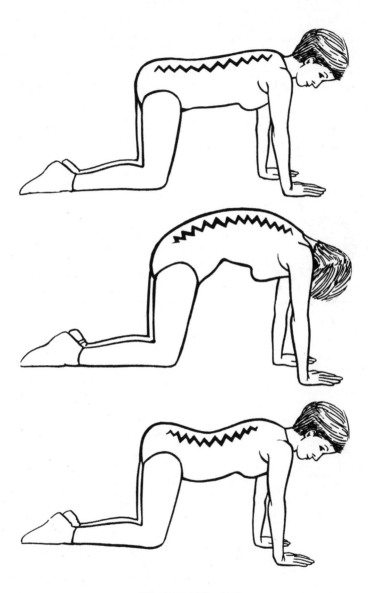

Figure 3.1 The Cat

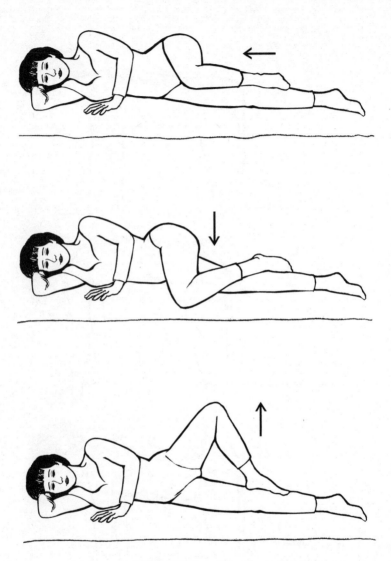

Figure 3.2 Knee Cross

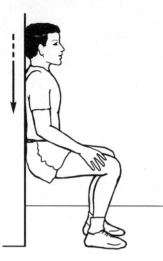

Figure 3.3 Wall Slide

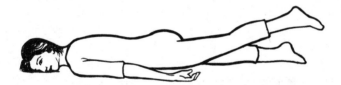

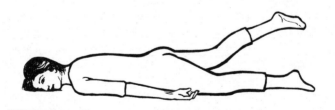

Figure 3.4 Leg Raises, Face Down

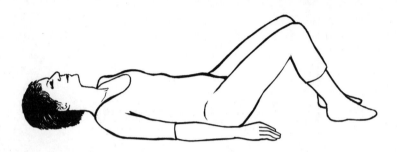

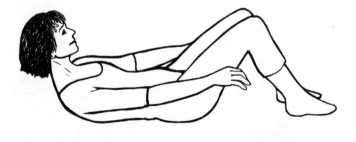

Figure 3.5 Mini Sit-up

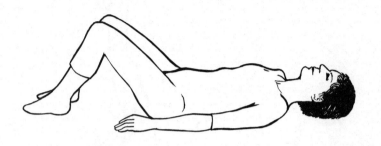

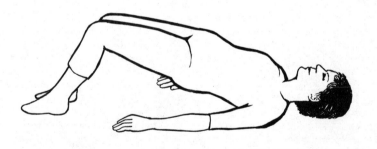

Figure 3.6 Pelvic Lift

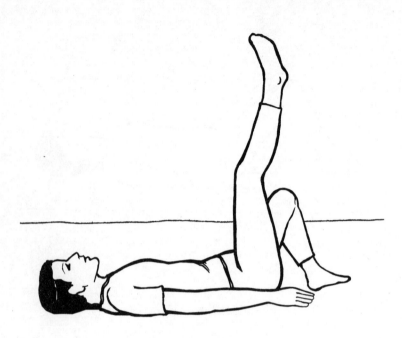

Figure 3.7 Leg Raises

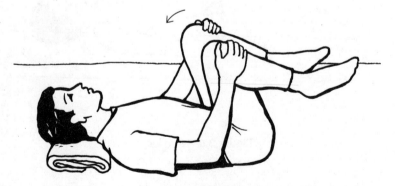

Figure 3.8 Roll Back

neck level, it's 90 percent. In water aerobics, you benefit from the resistance of the water, which means your muscles must work harder—and thus build strength and endurance—but there is minimal stress on the joints and spine.

Maggie's Story

Maggie had been suffering with chronic back pain for more than six months and was trying to control the pain with anti-inflammatory drugs and muscle relaxants. She thoroughly enjoyed her part-time job at a local book store, but standing on her feet for hours had gotten so painful she had to reduce her hours to less than fifteen per week. Her doctor referred her to a physical therapist, who did several massage sessions and developed a home exercise program for Maggie. After a few weeks, however, Maggie became discouraged with the exercises, saying they didn't work and were too painful, even though she was still taking anti-inflammatory medication. After she exhausted her insurance allowance for physical therapy, she lost all motivation to continue her exercise program and became depressed. One week after she stopped physical therapy, she quit her job.

Maggie's daughter, Sylvia, who lives in a neighboring state, visited her sixty-year-old mother and was concerned about her physical and mental condition. Sylvia had heard about water aerobics for chronic pain and asked her mother's doctor whether Maggie could safely participate. He said she could, and Sylvia immediately enrolled her mother in a water aerobics program for people who have back pain. The results, said Sylvia, were dramatic. "By the end of her second session, my mother was feeling better physically and emotionally," Sylvia said. "She discovered she could move with little or no pain.

She used to rate her pain an 8 out of 10, now she gave it a 2 or 3. Water aerobics gave her some control over her body and her pain, and she desperately needed that. It was a turning point for her."

Maggie's success with water aerobics improved her mood and allowed her to meet other people who were in situations similar to hers. Within a few weeks she began to socialize and decided to go back to work part-time. She was able to significantly reduce her use of medication as well.

Beginner's Water Aerobics

Here are three water aerobics exercises typically used in a beginner's program. These should be done in water that is chest- or above-the-waist high.

- **Walking in Water.** Begin at one end of the pool and walk across it as you would on land: swing your arms (in the water), keep your feet pointed straight ahead, and hold your head high. When you reach the other side, return by walking backward. This may be awkward at first, but take it slowly. When you walk backward, you use your hamstring and hip extensor muscles, which are very important for lower back stability. Keep your knees and legs straight, but if you feel some mild discomfort in your lower back, take smaller steps and bend your legs. If you feel a sharp or increased lower back or leg pain, stop walking backward and just do forward walking. Start your program by walking for several minutes and gradually increase the walking to eight to ten minutes per session.

- **Kicking in Water.** Stand perpendicular to the side of the pool and hold on to the side with your arm fully extended. Beginning with the leg that is farthest from the wall, raise it up as far as is comfortable, kick forward, and then bring it backward in one smooth motion and extend it behind you as far as is comfortable. Repeat the forward and backward kicks several times. Concentrate on keeping your back straight and your opposite leg straight, with your heel down. Do not lean forward or backward when you kick. When you have completed your kicks with that leg, turn around in the pool, hold on to the side again, and do the kicks with your other leg. Your goal is to eventually complete twenty-five to thirty kicks per leg at each session.

- **Side Kicks.** Stand in chest-high water perpendicular to the side of the pool and walk sideways by extending one leg to the side about shoulder width and then bringing your other leg to meet it. Keep repeating this movement until you reach the other side of the pool. If you prefer or if you need to hold on to the side of the pool, you can do this movement around the perimeter of the pool as long as the water is chest-high. When you reach a point where the water is higher or lower, simply reverse your steps. This exercise improves flexibility of the legs, hips, and trunk.

McKenzie Method

The McKenzie Method is a physical therapy approach that includes assessment, treatment, and prevention techniques, including exercises, that provide optimal benefits when they are learned with a qualified physical therapist. The goal of the physical therapist is to teach patients how to treat themselves and to minimize the risk of having recurring pain.

Although exercises are a big part of the McKenzie Method, the first step is a detailed assessment process, which patients need to go through so the physical therapist can select the most appropriate treatment plan. The assessment is based on the patient's pain history and responses to repeated test positions, movements, and activities that are done during the evaluation process that put the back either in extension (stretched backward) or flexion (arched forward). Once a patient's back pain has been classified, an appropriate treatment program can be arranged. Because everyone has a different response to the test, each person receives an individualized treatment plan.

The McKenzie Method is based on a very specific concept: that "centralizing" the pain allows the source of the pain, rather than the symptoms, to be treated. This approach is designed for patients who have back pain caused by an injured intervertebral disc, tears in the ligaments that surround a disc, or a herniated disc. The therapist chooses exercises that help extend the spine and arch the back, which in turn can reduce pressure on the offending disc(s). As the patient continues to do the exercises, the extensor muscles become stronger and help to "centralize" the damaged disc, thus reducing the amount of pressure on the ligaments in the back of the disc.

Patients typically see a physical therapist regularly for three to four weeks. The therapist can modify or replace exercises as a patient's pain decreases and range of motion increases. No ultrasound, medications, needles, heat, or cold are used.

Because of its centralizing focus, the McKenzie Method is not for everyone who has back pain. If your pain does not centralize, or if you have lumbar spinal stenosis or facet joint osteoarthritis, extending your spine may increase your pain. Certified McKenzie Method clinicians and your physician can identify whether you can benefit from the program or if you have a condition that is not suited for the treatment, and then prescribe the appropriate McKenzie exercises for you. After an initial education and treatment process, most patients can treat themselves at home. To find a certified McKenzie Method practitioner or clinic or for more information, see the resources section.

Dynamic Lumbar Stabilization Exercises

Your doctor and physical therapist may introduce you to an exercise technique called dynamic lumbar stabilization, a program that consists of eighty-four different exercises. The exercises are designed to retrain and strengthen the small muscles of the spine (proprioceptive muscles) that allow the spine to stay in a neutral spine position, which I talk about in chapter 4 under the discussion of Pilates. (Briefly, a neutral spine is aligned naturally and not flattened out.) Because your specific needs and condition differ from those of any other individual who has chronic low back pain, your therapist will individualize your exercise program to match those needs. The therapeutic program will consist of exercises at varying difficulty levels, and your therapist will work with you each step of the way as you progress through the program. It typically takes about six weeks to progress through the levels, and then a maintenance program is selected. Regular practice of these exercises results in improved strength in the torso, abdominal, and low back muscles and relief from pain.

Because dynamic lumbar stabilization exercises can be rigorous, they are not for everyone, especially if you have severe back pain or are physically frail. But they have proven to be very helpful for many people, including patients who have undergone surgery for a herniated lumbar disc. In an eight-week study that compared dynamic lumbar stabilization with a conventional home exercise program and no exercise at all, the investigators found that improvement among the patients who practiced dynamic lumbar stabilization exercises was highly significant compared with the other two groups, and that these specialized exercises relieved pain, improved function, and strengthened the abdominal, trunk, and lower back muscles.

Alexander Technique

The Alexander Technique is a method that teaches individuals how to be aware of the connection between their mind and body and, in that awareness, how to replace unhealthy, dysfunctional movements with healthier ones. Some people have called it mindfulness meditation brought to consciousness, because you are shown how everyday movements that you do unconsciously, such as picking up the newspaper from the driveway, reaching for something off a high shelf, or walking, if they are done inefficiently, can result in muscle tension, poor posture, fatigue, and inflexibility, all of which can contribute to and cause low back pain. Although there are few scientifically controlled studies of the effectiveness of the Alexander Technique for people who have chronic back pain, those that do exist support its use, while anecdotal reports are much more numerous.

The founder of the Alexander Technique, F. Matthias Alexander, said that the main purpose of the method is to "maintain the poise of the head on top of the lengthening spine in movement and at rest." In other words, good posture is much more than just standing up straight, it's about maintaining a stance in which the neck is free, the head is up, and the spine and torso are aligned and lengthened, both when you're moving and when you're not.

Alexander Technique teachers usually work one-on-one with students in sessions that last thirty to sixty minutes. At your first session, the teacher will evaluate your specific needs by asking questions about your activities, the type of work you do, and what you would like to accomplish. If there are certain activities or repetitive movements that may be contributing to your pain—for example, if your job requires you to reach overhead or to lift or turn—you may want to have the teacher evaluate those actions and help you learn better ways to move.

The teacher's task is to help you unlearn harmful habits and select new ones to incorporate into your lifestyle. The Alexander Technique is not an exercise program, so your teacher won't send you home with a list of exercises to do. You will, however, be expected to focus your attention on how you move throughout the day. The more conscious you are of your movements, the more likely your subconscious and your muscles are to be reprogrammed to adopt the new movements you learn from your teacher.

You can evaluate your posture to help you decide if the Alexander Technique is a treatment option for you. To do so, stand unclothed in front of a full-length mirror and objectively answer the following questions. If you answer yes to two or more of these questions, you may want to consider trying the Alexander Technique.

Front View:
- Does my chin extend too far forward?
- Do I cock my head to one side or the other?
- Do I extend my neck too far forward?
- Do I hunch my shoulders?
- Is one shoulder higher than the other?
- Are my shoulders rounded forward?

- Do I draw in my chest?
- Is one hip higher than the other?
- Do my arms hang evenly at my sides?

Side View
- Do I overarch my back?
- Does my stomach protrude?
- Do I hold my buttocks in too tight?
- Do I suck in my stomach?

If you think the Alexander Technique may help you, you should discuss the possibility with your health-care practitioner. See the resources section for more information.

Feldenkrais Method

The Feldenkrais Method was developed in the 1940s by an atomic research engineer who recognized through his own experiences with pain and injury that people have movement patterns that involve unnecessary muscle tension and that everyone can learn new ways to move that are gentle and graceful. It is a form of body education that consists of thousands of exercises taught by trained practitioners, who use a combination of these movements along with one-on-one manipulation. Through the Feldenkrais Method, you can gradually improve your posture, enhance your flexibility and coordination, increase your range of motion, and learn to move more efficiently and with less pain.

Joanne's Story

The road to the Feldenkrais Method was a long one for Joanne, who was the director of a large mental health organization. In 2000, at sixty-one years young, she had already experienced several lower back episodes, but each time she had bounced back within a few weeks. So when she bent down to lift a boom box from the floor and "threw her back out," she wasn't terribly concerned. But when the pain, which was "pretty awful," persisted for six weeks with no sign of letting up, she visited her general practitioner, who took X-rays, found nothing amiss, and told her she had spinal stenosis.

By then Joanne was finding it increasingly difficult to work. "Walking, sitting, standing—every position except lying curled up on my side was very painful," she said. A colleague suggested she see a chiropractor, which she did. She had some relief until the morning after her fifth session, when she woke up and couldn't move. That's when she decided to stop going to the chiropractor and take a leave of absence from her job to contemplate her next move. That move ended up being a visit to a rheumatologist, who ordered a CT scan and recommended physical therapy and a discectomy. Joanne made arrangements to begin physical therapy and decided against the surgery. At the end of six weeks of physical therapy, however, she felt little improvement.

Feeling discouraged, she followed up on a recommendation from the physical therapist to visit a physiatrist. She then underwent two series of epidural injections, which provided relief for several months each time, but offered no long-term solution. She then went to a neurosurgeon, who suggested a laminectomy. Again, she elected to forgo surgery and instead went to a pain clinic, started physical therapy, and had another series of epidural injections, which allowed her to return to work.

By now it was nearly two years since the "boom box" episode, and Joanne was still in pain, although able to work. She felt she had run out of options until a cousin told her how the Feldenkrais Method had helped a friend who had suffered for years with chronic low back pain. Joanne discovered that there was a Feldenkrais teacher not far from her home, and she made an appointment. At about the same time, Joanne made an appointment to see me for the first time. I strongly encouraged her to do the Feldenkrais and suggested she do a series of percutaneous electrical nerve stimulation (PENS) treatments to complement it. She completed a nine-treatment course of PENS, which she says relaxed her muscles enough so she could truly benefit from the Feldenkrais.

As of this writing, it is five years since Joanne picked up that boom box and three since she was introduced to Feldenkrais. She continues to visit her Feldenkrais teacher once a week and has "great posture" and minimal pain. She takes an anti-inflammatory and gabapentin (Neurontin) once a day, which is a far cry from the various opioids she was taking until she came to see me and we weaned her off them. She has a cane that she says "I don't really need but is great for getting a good parking spot and a seat on the train" and plans to continue seeing her teacher "as long as he can stand to see me."

Feldenkrais work is done in two ways. One is group classes, called Awareness Through Movement, in which the teacher verbally leads you through movements in such basic positions as standing or sitting. In private lessons, called Functional Integration, the movements are tailored to your specific needs, and the teacher guides your movements through touch.

Many Feldenkrais movements are done on a padded table or on the floor. Each movement is done slowly and gently and is designed to help increase your awareness of your body and how it communicates with your brain. The number of lessons you will need will depend on the severity of your pain and your physical condition, although, like Joanne, you can always keep going to sessions for follow-up or support. See the resources section for the location of Feldenkrais teachers in your area.

PHYSICAL THERAPY

For people who have chronic low back pain, physical therapy is a cornerstone of treatment and prevention, and when it is implemented by a good physical therapist, you've got a winning combination. The role of the therapist is to evaluate and implement a back treatment and prevention program that meets your specific needs and goals. Based on your criteria, the program may include ways to increase muscle strength and flexibility, improve range of motion and balance, and reduce pain. These goals can be accomplished in many ways, including a home exercise program, ultrasound, electrical stimulation, heat and/or ice, water aerobics, and various hands-on therapies (e.g., massage and manual manipulation).

The important thing to keep in mind is that exercise is the *primary* treatment tool in physical therapy, and the main task of the physical therapist is to identify, introduce, and help you develop the best exercise and movement program for you to achieve your goals. Other methods the physical therapist may use (e.g., ultrasound and massage) complement that program. Naturally, a physical therapist cannot make you do your exercises, so your full cooperation and participation are needed as well. In this section, we focus on the approaches your physical therapist may use to enhance your exercise program.

Physicians who see patients with back pain often work closely with one or more physical therapists and/or a pain management clinic or back program and offer referrals. If your doctor does not provide a referral or you want to find your own physical therapist, there are organizations that can help you locate some in your area (see the resources section).

Making Temperature Work for You

The application of heat and/or cold (cryotherapy) can be helpful for temporary reduction of inflammation and pain, especially when you first start an exercise program. Generally, heat improves blood circulation, reduces muscle spasm, improves tissue elasticity, and can cause or worsen inflammation. Heat should not be used if your tissues are inflamed or immediately after trauma. Cold reduces blood circulation and muscle spasm, decreases inflammation, numbs a site, and provides temporary pain relief.

Superficial heat, like that provided by a heating pad, hot water bottle, gel or clay pack, or liquid sodium acetate container can produce heating effects up to two centimeters, which is deep enough to help decrease muscle spasms and help make your exercise efforts less painful or stressful. Deeper tissues are usually protected against superficial heat because subcutaneous fat insulates them from the heat source, and increased blood flow in the skin dissipates the heat. Heat can be applied before and/or after each exercise session, as needed. Do not use heat therapy if you have diabetes unless you get approval from your doctor, and never go to sleep while using a heating device.

You will likely get more pain relief from cold than you will from heat. Ice or cold packs can reduce intramuscular temperatures by 3 to 7 degrees Celsius, which is enough to reduce local metabolism, inflammation, and pain. Cryotherapy works by reducing the velocity of pain signals along nerve fibers and decreasing muscle activity that is responsible for muscle tone. Cold packs are often used after a physical therapy or home exercise session to reduce pain and inflammation. Cold (not ice) packs can be applied over the affected area for fifteen to twenty minutes, three to four times a day initially, and then as needed. If you are applying ice packs, never place them directly against the skin, as the ice can freeze tissue. Ice packs typically come with a cover, which you should keep on the pack while in use. If the ice pack does not have a cover, place a thin, damp towel on the skin and put the ice pack on top of it. Do not use an ice pack for longer than ten minutes per treatment. Another approach, which can be helpful for the treatment of painful flares, is to alternate the use of ice and heat on the affected area.

You may find it helpful to wear a soft back brace with pockets that can hold hot and cold packs, or use thermal wraps, which usually contain gel packs that can be microwaved or frozen, thus allowing you to use them for heat or cold. These items can be found in medical supply stores and online.

Ultrasound

Ultrasound is a deep heating technique in which a device that emits high-frequency sound waves is passed over the affected area. These waves penetrate into the soft tissues and cause the molecules in the tissues to vibrate and produce heat. This in turn reportedly helps relieve pain, enhance tissue healing, and improve distensibility of connective tissue. The lower the frequency, the deeper the waves penetrate into the body. Your therapist can also vary the amount of heat by changing the frequency from intermittent to continuous.

There are conflicting reports on the effectiveness of ultrasound in the treatment of chronic low back pain. Some patients find ultrasound to be an effective complement when they first begin their exercise program, as it makes it easier and less painful for them to do stretching and other exercises, while others report little or no benefit. Ultrasound should not be used if you have inflammation, as it can make such conditions worse, or if you are pregnant.

Hydrotherapy

Hydrotherapy (also called water therapy) is one of the oldest therapeutic forms and one of the therapies that falls into both the active and passive categories. On the active side is water aerobics, which I discussed previously in this chapter. On the passive side are choices such as soaking in a warm bath or enjoying a sauna, whirlpool, or steam bath. Although these options do not provide major relief, they do increase circulation, loosen tense muscles, and help reduce stress, all of which are a welcome complement to other steps you take. Some patients find that hydrotherapy after an exercise session is a special treat.

If you are pregnant or if you have diabetes, high blood pressure, or a heart condition, make sure you consult with your doctor before you try any hydrotherapy options that may cause you to overheat, dehydrate, or experience undue stress.

Traction

Traction is a treatment method that involves the use of pulleys, weights, harnesses, flexing tables, and gravity to pull and stretch the muscles and ligaments to relieve disc or spinal alignment problems. For example, traction on the lower back is sometimes used to treat a herniated nucleus pulposus, which is the jellylike center of the disc. In this case, traction stretches the spine enough so the protruded disc can return to its normal or near normal position. Generally, a goal of each treatment is to relax the muscles and other support tissues and to relieve pain, not cause additional discomfort. Yet some people still think that traction involves torturous contraptions, when in fact it is a gentle way to relieve tension and pressure in the spine and increase circulation.

In-hospital traction is not used as much as it used to be, as it is usually not cost effective, given the high cost of medical care. However, short-term, outpatient traction can be a valuable complement to other ongoing treatments for chronic low back pain. Chiropractors, for example, frequently use a flexing table that allows them to gently traction the spine and release nerve pressure between segments of the vertebrae. Another type of traction occurs when a physical therapist assists a patient as he or she pulls on a harness that helps stretch the lower back.

Traction is not for everyone. If you have osteoporosis, cardiovascular disease, a hernia, fracture, or if you are pregnant, you should avoid spinal traction. A word of caution about home traction devices, including gravity-inversion traction: consult your doctor before attempting to use any such equipment. Traction should always be monitored by a knowledgeable health-care practitioner.

Massage

Soft tissue massage is often offered by physical therapists and licensed massage therapists as a way to loosen and relax the muscles, solely as therapy or as preparation for an exercise session. One of the most effective massage techniques for people who have chronic low back pain is myofascial massage, also known as myofascial release therapy. In this therapy method, which I discuss in more detail in chapter 4, the therapist uses gentle, kneading manipulation to stretch, soften, lengthen, and realign the fascia (the fibrous bands of connecting tissue). Your physical therapist may use this form of massage, or another type, before an exercise session to loosen and lengthen your muscles.

TENS

Transcutaneous electrical nerve stimulation (TENS) is a therapeutic technique that provides varying results for people who have low back pain. Although I cannot recommend TENS as a lone treatment for chronic low back pain, it can complement an exercise program and other treatments you may be pursuing. For some patients, it offers greater freedom of movement and an opportunity to more comfortably do their exercises, and so it is an asset for as long as it is effective. Unfortunately, the benefits of TENS do fade over time, and that amount of time varies with each person.

Keeping those caveats in mind, let's look at how TENS operates. A TENS device is a small (playing card–size), battery-powered unit that transmits mild electric pulses to nerve fibers, which in turn block incoming pain signals from the peripheral nerves on their way to the brain. The electrical pulses are delivered through electrodes that are placed at or near painful areas on the body. TENS may also help stimulate the production of the body's natural pain-relieving substances, endorphins, in the brain. It is a safe therapy that patients who have not had success with medication or who want to avoid it, people who are recovering from back surgery, and those with sciatica might want to consider. TENS is most useful for individuals whose source of back pain is a single nerve root, as is pain caused by shingles.

If you and your doctor decide a TENS unit may help you, he or she must prescribe it for you, but a physical therapist, nurse, or other trained health-care professional can work with you to explain how to use the unit and monitor your progress. The TENS unit can be clipped to your belt or placed in a pocket, and the lead wires with electrodes can be placed under your clothing to the treatment sites. The closer the electrodes are to the offending nerves, the lower the current needed to stimulate the nerve fibers. Often it takes several attempts to find the most effective spots to place the electrodes, so expect a trial-and-error period.

When you turn the unit on, a low level of electricity travels through the electrodes and stimulates the nerve fibers, blocking the pain signals to the brain. Some patients feel a slight tingling sensation when the unit is on; others say they don't feel anything unusual. You may feel relief from pain immediately, or it may take hours, although twenty minutes is the average time for benefits to become apparent. The level of relief and how long it lasts vary from patient to patient: some experience relief for hours after they turn the device off, while others only get relief while the unit is on.

The advantages of a TENS unit, however, are that it is safe, and you have control over when you get treatment, the length of the treatment, and the intensity of the stimulation. All units allow you to adjust the intensity of the stimulation, and some have the added feature of letting you select high- or low-frequency stimulation. High-frequency stimulation tends to cause little or no unusual sensations and so is easily tolerated for hours, but the resulting pain relief lasts for a shorter time than that provided by low-frequency stimulation, which can result in tingling and minor discomfort and lead users to turn the unit off after twenty to thirty minutes. However, pain relief is usually longer lasting with low-frequency stimulation.

One drawback in recommending TENS for chronic low back pain is that there are few well-controlled studies evaluating its efficacy. In one study, TENS was compared with massage in people with low back pain, and TENS was significantly more effective in decreasing pain. In yet another study, in which patients with job-related injuries received TENS in long-term rehabilitation programs, 44 percent of patients were able to return to work after six months of therapy, and an additional 36 percent returned to work part-time. Overall, the patients experienced a decrease in pain, improved sleep, and a reduced need for pain medications because of TENS treatment.

A TENS-like stimulation therapy called interferential current therapy (ICT) sends out a higher frequency than a TENS unit, and thus the waves penetrate the skin more deeply and result in less user discomfort. ICT is more effective in treating muscle spasm and is very effective in treating chronic myofascial pain. Because the technology is more complex than that of TENS, the units are more expensive. In chapter 4, I discuss the use of TENS versus PENS, a type of acupuncture. Although PENS appears to be more effective than TENS, the latter remains a viable option for patients who want the freedom to treat themselves. The only side effect of note is that long-term stimulation of the same electrode sites can irritate the skin of some people. TENS is not recommended for people who are pregnant, who have a demand-type cardiac pacemaker, or who have heart disease or epilepsy.

PHYSICAL SUPPORTS

Many physicians overlook the use of physical supports to reduce stress on the lumbar spine; yet braces, corsets, orthotics, and other devices can be instrumental in reducing pain. In most cases, the use of physical supports is only a temporary measure, necessary only as long as it takes to restore strength or range of motion, or to facilitate rehabilitation or recovery from a medical procedure.

Orthotics

When you stand and walk, your lumbar spine and pelvis balance on your hips and legs. If you have alignment problems with your hips, legs, or feet, an abnormal amount of force can be transmitted to your spine. For example, if you have degenerative lumbar discs and facets, your heel may not align with the ground when you step down. When you consider that every step you take is misaligned, each step can send undue stress to the spine and contribute to low back pain. Some of this force can be reduced significantly with the use of custom-made orthotics that fit easily and comfortably into your shoes. Orthotics or heel lifts can also help if you have a difference in leg length, a condition that produces abnormal strain on the lower back and pelvis and even results in degenerative changes to the spine.

Yet for some patients, orthotics seem to open up a Pandora's box. Patients who have had a lifelong leg length discrepancy, for example, may experience problems with balance and biomechanics once they add lift to their shoes. Paula Breuer explains that an orthotic, when it is used to correct one problem, may place an abnormal amount of stress on a joint and unwittingly cause other problems. "If a patient has a sunken arch," she says, "he or she usually has a lot of joint stiffness. If a patient is prescribed an orthotic to correct the arch, it may suddenly place too much stress on another joint and cause the patient to have pain." At that point the patient decides to stop using the orthotic because it appears to be causing more pain instead of less. Thus, if you get a corrective device such as orthotics, your doctor should be aware that he or she may need to make additional adjustments. If you are considering orthotics, you might consider trying over-the-counter orthotics, and if they provide some relief, then you may want to get custom-made orthotics. Before you do anything, however, discuss your options with a physical therapist.

Braces, Belts, and Corsets

Although braces, belts, and corsets may seem like an old-fashioned way to approach back pain, they can be helpful in certain situations. Generally, these devices help avoid undesirable movement, assist with proper posture, reduce weight-bearing stress on the spine, and stabilize the lower back. After surgery for spinal fusion or fractures, for example, motion of the lower spine can delay proper healing, while wearing a brace temporarily can speed up the healing process as well as decrease low back pain and discomfort.

Two types of braces are available: rigid braces, which are made of form-fitting plastic and can limit approximately 50 percent of motion in the spine; and elastic braces (corset braces), which are rarely recommended after a lumbar fusion, as there is limited evidence that soft braces are very effective in stabilizing the lumbar spine. Corset braces prevent you from bending forward and are sometimes used by people who do a lot of heavy lifting.

Short-term use of a corset brace is also helpful if your back muscles are fatigued or irritated because of a recent injury. Some braces have adjustable air-pressure bladders that place direct pressure over irritated areas, and this can provide significant relief and be helpful during the initial part of your recovery. Wearing a back brace for a prolonged period, however, can contribute to weakened back muscles. Once an injury has healed sufficiently, the best rule of thumb is to use a back brace only if your spine needs protection against an activity, such as lifting and moving heavy objects.

A sacroiliac belt (SI belt) helps stabilize the SI joint and reduces strain on the ligaments of the joint. It is sometimes helpful for people who have hypermobility of the sacroiliac joint following trauma or childbirth. An SI belt is also useful for individuals who engage in certain activities, especially job-related, that can strain the SI joint, such as those that require pushing or pulling.

IN CONCLUSION . . .

In the vast majority of cases, physical exercise is the most effective treatment for chronic low back pain. An exercise program should be designed to meet your specific strengths, weaknesses, and physical condition and allow you to participate as fully as possible in your normal lifestyle activities. It also should serve as the foundation from which you can add complementary therapies, such as those offered by a physical therapist, as discussed in this chapter, or various mind-body options, such as those discussed in the next two chapters. Patients who stay with an exercise program often find that their quality of life—physically, emotionally, and mentally—improves and that they are able to ward off or be better prepared for any future episodes of back pain.

Chapter 4

Step 2: Body Therapies

When patients who have chronic back pain include gentle body therapies as part of their healing program, they often reap very significant benefits. Men and women have told me repeatedly how incorporating such techniques as acupuncture, chiropractic, massage, Pilates, tai chi, and yoga has significantly improved the quality of their lives.

"Acupuncture and yoga gave me my life back," says Karla, a forty-nine-year-old waitress at a tennis resort. Although she says her chronic pain seemed to "come out of nowhere," she knows that the long hours on her feet on the job and carrying banquet trays had taken their toll on her back over the years. Karla tried various anti-inflammatory and muscle-relaxing drugs, but she wasn't pleased with the results or the drugs' side effects. She was exhausted from fighting the pain and the adverse reactions, and she had no energy to do much else after work.

One of Karla's customers, a massage therapist, suggested she try massage and offered her two free sessions to see how she liked it. Karla calls it "the best tip I ever got. I noticed some relief after the first session." When the therapist recommended yoga as a complement to the massage therapy, Karla didn't need any prodding. Now she practices yoga every day and gets a "booster" massage once a month. "I don't need the drugs anymore," says Karla, "and I even took up swimming. Massage and yoga have made a big difference in my life."

I have witnessed how many patients with chronic low back pain have benefited from trying various body therapies and heard the enthusiasm in their voices when they tell me about the relief they receive. Increasingly, data from numerous research studies support their claims as well. So I want to share these options with you. In this chapter, we explore natural body-based therapies that you can use along with other approaches discussed in part II. I offer guidelines on how you can incorporate these techniques into your life and provide resources for finding practitioners. I also discuss how to choose the best lifestyle devices to help support body therapies, such as mattresses, ergonomic chairs, and other items that support the back and help prevent pain and further injury.

ACUPUNCTURE

In 2001, I became a licensed medical acupuncturist and joined the growing number of physicians who have embraced this traditional Chinese healing method. According to traditional Chinese medicine, acupuncture is based on the theory that pain and disease occur when the body's natural energy force, or *chi*, is out of balance. This life force travels throughout the body along channels called *meridians*, and one way its flow can be influenced (stimulated or altered) at specific points (acupoints) along those channels is through the use of very fine acupuncture needles. Stimulation of certain acupoints can correct the blocked or improper flow of chi, which in turn can bring relief from pain or disease.

How Acupuncture Works: The Science

The reasons acupuncture benefits at least some patients who are in pain are not entirely clear. Most experts believe that the insertion of the needles stimulates the central nervous system and results in the release of specific chemicals such as endorphins, which are the body's natural painkillers and which can play a critical role in breaking the cycle of pain. One benefit of acupuncture is that it can be used along with other treatments, including medication, and can reduce the need for medications and their adverse effects.

Although acupuncture was once regarded with much skepticism by the majority of conventional medical professionals, it is now earning some much-deserved respect among mainstream practitioners. In 1998, in fact, the National Institutes of Health (NIH) issued a statement in which it said that in certain situations, including back pain, acupuncture "may be useful as an adjunct treatment or an acceptable alternative or be included in a comprehensive management program." The NIH also concluded that further research was needed before a more solid endorsement could be made.

I, along with many other researchers, share that opinion as well. In a 2005 issue of the *Annals of Internal Medicine*, for example, investigators reported on their review of approximately two dozen previously published studies of acupuncture. They concluded that acupuncture is "significantly more effective" than no treatment in people who have chronic back pain. At the same time, the investigators also reported that the number of studies available for review is "limited in quantity and quality." The consensus is that we need controlled studies that include a great number of patients and are conducted over a long period of time. In fact, at least one such study has been done.

In a two-year follow-up study conducted at the University of Sheffield in England, researchers evaluated 239 patients ages eighteen to sixty-five who had chronic low back pain: 159 received up to ten acupuncture treatments and 80 received traditional care (medication) from their general practitioners. After both twelve and twenty-four months, patients who had received acupuncture treatments were significantly more likely to report being pain-free and much less likely to use medication than those who had taken medication only.

PENS: A Different Type of Acupuncture

Although traditional Chinese acupuncture can be quite helpful for people who have acute back pain, I find it to be less effective for those who have chronic pain. However, a form of acupuncture called percutaneous electrical nerve stimulation (PENS) (a special type of electroacupuncture) is very helpful in treating chronic low back pain.

When using PENS to treat chronic low back pain, as with traditional acupuncture, fine needles are placed in the muscles or soft tissues at specific points. The needles are attached to a device that transmits continuous low-intensity electrical impulses. PENS differs from traditional Chinese electroacupuncture in that with PENS, needles are placed according to the arrangement of the spinal nerves and the muscles they feed, whereas traditional Chinese acupuncture guides needle placement using the system of meridians.

Again and again, I've seen how effective PENS can be. Rosalind, a sixty-nine-year-old retired secretary, readily agrees. When she first came to see me, she had been suffering with low back pain as well as left leg pain and paresthesia (tingling and numbness) for six months. Except for high blood pressure, which she had largely controlled with exercise and diet, she was in good health. The pain, she said, had "come out of nowhere" and had worsened quickly. Before that time, Rosalind had taken great joy in walking three miles a day around the lake near her home, but now she could barely walk for ten minutes before the pain became too much to bear. She was worried not only about her back and leg pain but about not being able to exercise properly to control her blood pressure.

Her previous doctor had ordered an MRI, which showed spinal stenosis. He then prescribed physical therapy, which consisted of massage, heat, and a home exercise program, but Rosalind had not gotten much relief, even when she added anti-inflammatory medication. She then agreed to undergo epidural corticosteroid injections, but they provided only modest, temporary relief.

Based on my experience with PENS (see PENS: The Research), I felt that Rosalind was a good candidate for the therapy. When I explained PENS to Rosalind, she said, "I need to get back on my feet. Let's go for it." Initially I treated her once a week for four weeks, and then gradually reduced treatments to one every three months. Today Rosalind is back strolling around the lake. She shuns any anti-inflammatory medication and has managed thus far to stay away from antihypertensive drugs as well. I've also encouraged her to reintroduce back exercises into her daily routine and to consider tai chi to help maintain balance.

I have also had some success using PENS with people who have come to me with failed back surgery syndrome (FBSS), a condition I discuss in more detail in chapter 8. As the name indicates, people with FBSS have not gotten relief from their back surgery. PENS can be an effective alternative, especially when individuals are faced with the possibility of undergoing another surgery. One drawback to this idea, however, is that many insurers will not pay for PENS, which means patients must pay for it out-of-pocket.

PENS: The Research

In 2003, my colleagues and I published a pilot study on the use of PENS in thirty-four older adults who had chronic low back pain. In the six-week study, half the patients received PENS and physical therapy, and half received sham PENS (just the needles without electrical stimulation) and physical therapy. After six weeks and again after an additional three months, the patients who had received PENS reported a significant reduction in pain intensity and disability, as well as significant improvement in physical performance, mood, and life control. None of these results were true for the sham-PENS patients. The success of this study prompted us to do another. I am now conducting a large, randomized, controlled trial of PENS to be completed in 2007.

Several other studies have provided much promising support for the use of PENS in chronic low back pain. In Hong Kong, for example, Dr. C. K. Yeung and his colleagues found that a combination of PENS and back exercises is an effective treatment option for relief of pain and disability in people with chronic low back pain. A recent (2004) Japanese study looked at eighteen patients with chronic low back pain who underwent twice-weekly treatments with PENS for eight weeks, while another seventeen patients received PENS for four weeks and then TENS (in which electric current is delivered through the skin) for four weeks. A third group of eighteen received TENS for eight weeks.

Overall, the investigators found that patients in the PENS-only group experienced significant pain relief from week 2 of treatment that continued up to one month after treatment ended. This was not true for the other two treatment groups. By the second month after the end of PENS treatment, however, the pain-relief advantage had disappeared. The researchers concluded, therefore, that PENS is more effective than TENS for chronic low back pain and that the pain-relieving benefit lasts for several weeks after treatment ends, which means patients need regular treatments to sustain pain relief. My own experience with PENS has shown me that the duration of pain relief is variable. Some patients can go for several months between treatments.

Is Acupuncture for You?

"I can't believe it didn't hurt." That's what many patients say after they've had their first acupuncture session. Acupuncture needles are very thin, almost hairlike, and their insertion does not feel like you're getting an injection from your doctor. In fact, many people find they can relax and even fall asleep during treatment once their initial anxiety is put to rest.

If you are considering acupuncture, look for a licensed and accredited professional who will answer your questions and who makes you feel at ease. Some medical doctors, like myself, are certified in acupuncture and have experience working with patients who have back pain. If you need help finding an acupuncture practitioner in your area, consult your physician or local hospital, or see the resources section for the names of referring organizations.

CHIROPRACTIC

The concept behind chiropractic, that the body has the ability to heal itself once the central nervous system—and the spinal vertebrae that protect it—is in alignment, makes it a viable treatment option for individuals whose back pain is associated with misaligned vertebrae. These out-of-place bones can put pressure on nearby nerves and cause a condition called subluxation, which a chiropractor may correct using various spinal manipulative therapy techniques, such as acupressure, massage, or other types of body manipulation. Among these manipulations is the practice of "cracking" the back, a practice that sounds much more ominous than it really is. When a chiropractor, osteopath, or other specially trained medical professional "cracks" your back or neck, he or she is moving a joint past the point where it usually goes (called the passive range of motion) but not past the point where it can move safely. The "crack" or popping is the sound made when gases are released within the joint fluid when the joint is moved.

Being "Activated"

Another chiropractic approach is the use of an activator, a stick-shaped device that delivers light, measured force to the site to which it is applied. The force is a gentle, painless way to realign vertebrae. Vivian, a sixty-three-year-old retired history teacher, says she was skeptical when she first went to a chiropractor for relief of lower back and leg pain she had had for several years following an automobile accident. "I was tired of the pain and tired of the pills," she says. "When I started to get tingling in my right arm, I decided I had had enough. A friend recommended her chiropractor, who had helped her after a fall down some stairs. The chiropractor used something called an activator, and after just two treatments, not only was my arm better, but my lower back pain improved. After several more treatments I stopped taking the NSAIDs [nonsteroidal anti-inflammatory drugs], and now I find that I only need them on rare occasions. That was more than two years ago."

Vivian still visits her chiropractor about twice a year for what she calls "tweaking," and she starts and ends each day with ten minutes of stretching exercises that he recommended. She also walks two miles with a neighbor several times a week and recently started taking ballroom dance lessons. "If there's one thing I learned about back pain it's that you can't be passive about it," Vivian says. "Get help, get moving, and you'll get better."

Going to a Chiropractor

The type of treatments you can expect from a chiropractor will depend on the type of chiropractor you choose. Straight chiropractors, which comprise about 15 percent of all chiropractors, focus on spinal manipulations and subluxation. The majority of chiropractors are mixed, meaning they incorporate supplements, nutrition, mind-body techniques, homeopathy, and other therapies along with spinal manipulations as part of their treatment plan. Among these therapies are flexibility and strength exercises that are designed to improve the lumbar spine and decrease pain. We talked about various exercises and movement therapies in chapter 3, but here I want to mention the role chiropractors can play in this decision.

The type(s) of exercises that are best for your particular situation can be identified by your chiropractor if your physician and/or physical therapist have not already done so. It's important to follow an exercise plan that has been designed specifically for you. Don't use one recommended by a friend or that was put together for a family member.

To determine which exercises will best address your needs, a chiropractor will need to perform clinical testing and a postural evaluation, which you can expect on your first visit.

What to Expect

On your first visit, the chiropractor should gather medical history information and conduct a physical examination. If you have the results of any tests, including blood tests, urinalysis, X-rays, or other scans, you should bring those with you or have them sent from your physician's office. If you have no prior scan results and the chiropractor insists on ordering X-rays or an MRI, the same warning applies here as it does with your primary-care physician: X-rays and scans should be ordered only if there is evidence of obvious spinal problems. My personal recommendation, however, is that an individual's physician should decide whether a spinal X-ray or MRI is necessary, not a chiropractor, and that patients should seek the help of a chiropractor only after he or she has gotten permission from a primary-care physician.

The chiropractor will evaluate your muscle tone and strength and the range of motion in your spine and other joints, as well as conduct a neurological examination to test your coordination, reflexes, sensation, and vision. These evaluations are done while you stand, sit on the edge of an examining table, or lie on the table, and the main diagnostic technique he or she will use is palpation. Palpation is a technique of examining through touch, and it is one of the primary ways a chiropractor determines where and how to adjust the spine. One approach is static palpation, in which the chiropractor palpates the tissue that surrounds the spine, searching for tenderness, tightness, pain, and other indications of tissue injury. In motion palpation, the chiropractor examines each spinal joint and identifies any that lack the proper amount of motion.

Before starting any manipulations, your chiropractor may apply heat or ice or use massage to relax your muscles. Chiropractic care for chronic low back pain may require just a few treatments or, as one study shows, up to two to three weeks of daily manipulation. In a study of 238 patients who were completely disabled with chronic low back and leg pain that had not responded to previous traditional or surgical treatment, 81 percent experienced significant improvement after undergoing daily chiropractic manipulations for two to three weeks. Many patients find that a treatment every two to six months or longer, following a more intense series of manipulations for a month or two, maintains them at a significantly reduced level of pain.

Before I leave chiropractic, a quick caveat. Generally, chiropractic treatment, or any manual technique for that matter, is most effective when it is administered during the first four weeks after acute injury. Although many back pain patients seek care from chiropractors, there are no convincing studies of the effectiveness of chiropractic for relief of chronic low back pain. Despite this lack of evidence from controlled studies, a significant number of patients with chronic pain reports positive or satisfactory results, and so its value cannot be dismissed.

MASSAGE

One of the oldest and more effective ways to treat lower back pain is massage. Whether a massage is given by a licensed massage therapist or a caring partner (with some guidance), the benefits can be substantial. Recognition of the value of massage in the treatment of back pain is widespread, especially in

Europe. In Austria, for example, 87 percent of people with back pain receive massage as part of their conventional (not alternative) care. In the United States, massage has not reached that level of acceptance, but it is definitely growing in popularity. A study in the *Journal of the American Medical Association* reported that Americans visit a massage therapist more than 114 million times a year, especially for chronic conditions such as back pain and headache, while results of a national survey found that visits to massage therapists are increasing. People are going to massage therapists because they can reap some significant benefits. For example, massage can

- release tension in tight muscles, which in turn relieves pain
- increase blood and lymph circulation
- improve range of motion, which in turn can improve quality of life
- help rid the body of the toxic by-products of muscle metabolism, which contribute to pain
- increase endorphin levels. Endorphins are the body's natural painkillers. The body produces more of these chemicals during massage.

Body massage can have a soothing effect on your emotional and mental well-being as well. As one patient puts it, "When I get a massage for my back, my mind gets pain relief as well. I can feel the stress melt away while my muscles are being worked. It's like a mini vacation."

Proof Is in the Touch

Although massage can be helpful for lower back pain stemming from various causes, it can be especially beneficial for those who have myofascial pain, which commonly contributes to lower back pain. Many of my patients report feeling significantly better once they try massage, and scientific research supports their reports. In a study published in the *International Journal of Neuroscience* and conducted at the Touch Research Institute at the University of Miami in 2001, for example, the investigators noted that "massage lessened lower back pain, depression and anxiety. . . . The massage therapy group also showed improved range of motion, and their serotonin and dopamine [neurotransmitter] levels were higher." Neurotransmitters—chemicals found throughout the body, but especially in the brain—are associated with depression and are believed by some experts to play a major role in chronic pain.

Types of Massage

There are literally hundreds of different types of massage, but some of the more common ones in the United States are Swedish massage, acupressure, neuromuscular therapy, and myofascial release therapy.

Swedish massage is perhaps the most well recognized form in the United States. It combines a variety of techniques, including effleurage (slow, rhythmic stroking), kneading, pétrissage (forceful rolling of the skin), tapotement (percussive movements), vibration (shaking with both hands), and friction (application of pressure with the fingertips using circular motions). A licensed massage therapist should be proficient in all of these applications. It's a good idea to experience a professional massage so you know what a therapeutic massage can do for you. Unfortunately, many insurance plans do not cover the cost of this therapeutic option, and so the out-of-pocket cost of Swedish massage prevents some people from enjoying it.

But it isn't necessary to go to a professional. If you have a partner or friend who is willing to give you a massage, he or she can take several lessons or learn enough from an instructional video to help you. Consider taking a class in couples massage. If possible, occasionally schedule a massage with a professional.

Acupressure is a type of massage that is based on the same theory as acupuncture: acupoints along the energy channels (meridians) are the sites that need to be addressed during treatment. Whereas an acupuncturist uses needles, an acupressure therapist uses fingers, palms, and elbows to apply pressure to acupoints for several minutes to stimulate the flow of healing energy (chi). Shiatsu is an ancient Japanese massage that is based on acupressure.

I suggest going to a professional acupressure therapist for treatment. However, some patients learn some of the basic acupressure points and treat themselves or ask a partner or friend to help them, and they are pleased with the results. Ruth, a fifty-year-old journalist, did a little research on acupressure for sciatica and found several self-help books on the method. Now she routinely treats her chronic sciatic pain by applying pressure to selected acupoints. "I feel better within minutes of treating myself," she says. "The pain doesn't go away completely, but it's so much more bearable, and I can do the treatments wherever I am—in the car, while standing in line, or while working at the computer. And that's important to me, that I have control over my treatment."

Neuromuscular therapy has been recognized by the American Academy of Pain Management as an effective treatment for back pain that is caused by injury to the soft tissues, such as muscle strain and myofascial pain. In neuromuscular therapy, the therapist relaxes the muscles one layer at a time by working gently and slowly to completely release the tension in a more superficial layer of muscle before applying additional pressure and moving on to the next layer. The pressure is usually applied with the fingers, knuckles, or elbow and is held for about ten to thirty seconds. Muscles that are in spasm are painful to the touch, and the pain is caused by an insufficient flow of blood to the muscle, which means the muscle also is not receiving enough oxygen. A lack of oxygen causes muscles to produce lactic acid, which in turn makes muscles feel sore following activity. As the therapist applies pressure, the muscles relax, releasing lactic acid and allowing sufficient blood and oxygen to flow again. Neuromuscular therapy takes several sessions to accomplish—usually four to six, depending on the severity of the tension and pain. If you try to rush through therapy, the result may be more pain rather than less.

Although there is usually some pain associated with neuromuscular therapy itself, relief follows the initial discomfort. I encourage patients to communicate with their therapist about the amount of pressure he or she is using. In fact, many people say they feel a "good pain" during neuromuscular massage therapy. After each session, any soreness typically fades within twenty-four to thirty-six hours, and the muscles that were worked on should remain noticeably relaxed for days to weeks. You can help maintain that relaxed state by doing daily stretching exercises or other physical activities as recommended by your doctor or therapist, such as yoga, Pilates, tai chi, or water aerobics.

Myofascial release therapy is a technique in which gentle stretching is combined with massage to relieve pain and promote healing by improving posture, releasing tension, and increasing circulation, flexibility, and range of motion. This approach made its debut in the late 1970s, and since then it's been adopted by physical therapists, osteopaths, chiropractors, and other health-care professionals to help alleviate the chronic pain associated with back pain, fibromyalgia, sciatica, and neck pain.

Myofascial release therapy is based on the concept that poor posture, physical injury and trauma, and emotional stress can all cause the fascia (fibrous bands of connective tissue that are wrapped around muscles, nerves, bones, and blood vessels) throughout the body to constrict. This can occur when any of these sheaths of tissue are injured or strained, and the stress of these injuries causes painful adhesions or scar tissue to attach to muscle fibers. Eventually the pain can lead to limited movement and misalignment throughout the body, including the spine.

Many physical therapists offer myofascial release therapy because it is an effective technique to prepare the body for exercise sessions. Myofascial release therapists blend stretches and massage to ease pressure in the fascia, release the adhesions, lengthen the fascia, and help restore balance. Treatments typically involve very gentle stretching of muscles and connective tissue. Each stretch may be held for up to five minutes, until the therapist feels the tension "release." Because the fascia is an interconnected network, the therapist will likely do stretches on parts of your body that don't hurt but are indirectly contributing to the pain.

Therapy sessions usually last about thirty minutes and, depending on the severity of your condition, may be recommended several times a week for a month or two. In between sessions, you should practice stretches and exercises that have been given to you by your therapist.

Patients who try myofascial release therapy usually find that not only do they enjoy relief from pain, but they can also reduce or even eliminate their need for painkillers and muscle relaxants. An added benefit here, of course, is reduced or no exposure to the potentially dangerous side effects associated with drug use.

Is Massage for You?

Massage can be used to complement many of the other treatment options discussed in this book, and given the many different forms of massage therapy available, there may be something for everyone. But for one reason or another, massage may not be for you. Consider these guidelines when thinking about whether massage therapy should be part of your treatment plan.

- Consult your physician before choosing massage as a treatment for your back pain. Most massage therapists are not medical doctors, so you need to learn from your doctor whether it is safe for you to get a massage and what type of massage therapy would be safe for you.
- Be aware that if your muscles are inflamed, massage isn't for you. You may fare better with water aerobics, hydrotherapy, and perhaps some anti-inflammatory medication. Also, if you have muscle spasms and you don't experience some improvement after two massage treatments, massage may not be the best choice for you.
- Pay attention to the contraindications for massage, which include the presence of phlebitis, open wounds, severe osteoporosis, deep vein thrombosis, eczema, fractures, and burns. If you are pregnant, some stretches or movements may not be appropriate.
- Drink lots of water during or after each session. Water helps flush out toxins from the body and relieve any soreness you may experience after your massage.

PILATES

Pilates (pronounced *pi-LAH-teez*) is a form of exercise that focuses on the core postural muscles that provide support for the spine. A key principle of Pilates is that of the neutral spine, and individuals who practice Pilates learn how to maintain it. A neutral spine is one that is ideally aligned, which means all four curves are in balance with each other and none are excessive: an inward curve in the cervical and lumbar regions, and an outward curve in the thoracic region and sacral spine. Pilates exercises are designed to strengthen the deep postural muscles that support this alignment.

Patients who have back pain that is caused by excessive movement and degeneration of the intervertebral discs and joints (e.g., degenerative disc disease) can especially benefit from a Pilates program. Pilates exercises can improve any asymmetry of posture, which in turn decreases wear and tear caused by uneven stress on the intervertebral joints and discs. They improve muscle strength, flexibility, and suppleness of muscles and joints, and also teach awareness of movement and posture habits that may be causing stress to the spine. As patients become aware of any negative habits they may have, including how they hold tension in their muscles, they can replace them with those that help preserve a neutral spine and a healthier back and improve well-being.

Georgia's Story

Georgia, a fifty-something social worker, was introduced to Pilates three decades after her original back injury, which occurred when someone slammed into her back while she and friends were on a mountain slide at an amusement park. At the time she consulted a neurologist because of the severe pain, which she treated with diazepam (Valium) and ice packs, and experienced limited movement for about two months. The pain gradually subsided, and for years she didn't experience any significant painful episodes, until her late thirties, when she lifted a lawn mower into the trunk of her car. The move left her in severe pain, which again gradually subsided but didn't go away. Despite lingering discomfort and compromised movement, Georgia said, "I had no choice; I had to work," and treated herself with ibuprofen.

The next few episodes occurred closer together—another painful bout caused by moving some boxes, and the latest one, five years ago, while shoveling snow. "The last injury was pretty bad," she said. "I couldn't move, and I knew it was time for me to take care of my back." During a visit to her family physician, Georgia was given muscle relaxants to manage her muscle spasms and was referred to a physical therapist. There she was introduced to Pilates.

Before she started learning and practicing Pilates, however, Georgia underwent ultrasound and took NSAIDs to alleviate the pain enough to allow her to begin exercise. The ultrasound and drugs have long since stopped, but Georgia continues practicing Pilates every day. "I know what happens if I don't exercise every day," she says. "I haven't had a severe spasm since I started Pilates. My pain level is very manageable, a 2 to 3 on a scale of 10. I love to garden, and working in the yard makes me aware of my back pain; but so does just getting out of bed." Georgia has since added a weekly session of Kripalu yoga to her program (see Yoga in this chapter) and is contemplating acupuncture to see if it can alleviate the lingering pain.

Is Pilates for You?

I have personally seen many patients benefit from Pilates, but it is not an exercise program for everyone. Pilates has its roots in dance and ballet, and so some of the movements can be challeng-ing for some people, although many of the exercises are simple and very accessible. Regardless of their complexity, it's critical that the exercises be learned and performed correctly, because those that are done incorrectly can make back pain worse.

Therefore, make sure your Pilates instructor has received formal Pilates training and that he or she is knowledgeable about your specific back problem. It is best to go to a Pilates instructor who has been recommended by a physical therapist or other health professional or, if you are fortunate, you will find a physical therapist who has had formal Pilates training. In any case, the instructor should help you develop an exercise program that will advance your rehabilitation. If you have sig-nificant back problems, you may want to work one-on-one with a Pilates instructor, at least for a few sessions, until you feel comfortable and confident that you understand how the exercises should be done. You can then move on to a group class. Weekly sessions may be sufficient if you practice exercises at home between sessions.

TAI CHI

Calm, slow, fluid, balancing, and flowing: these are words that are often used to describe tai chi, a form of exercise that is based on the ancient Chinese martial art of tai chi chuan. Rather than engaging in combative movements, however, tai chi exercise is a modification of the martial art. These modifi-cations embrace three components that form the foundation of tai chi and work to help heal the body. They are

- movement: All movements are fluid, slow, and deliber-ate. They help improve posture, spine alignment (the neutral spine talked about in the section on Pilates), strength, balance, coordination, flexibility, range of motion, and endurance.

- meditation: Participants in tai chi are encouraged to assume a meditative state of mind, which, along with the fluid movements and breathing (see below), helps eliminate anxiety, tension, and stress, all of which contribute to and enhance pain.
- breathing: The proper practice of tai chi includes focused, rhythmic breathing that promotes good circulation and delivers much-needed oxygen to the muscles, which in turn helps relieve pain.

The Benefits of Tai Chi

Most people use their body incorrectly. They practice poor posture, lift improperly, slouch, wear damaging shoes, sleep on poor mattresses, and don't exercise nearly enough. Tai chi is a wonderful discipline, because it helps its practitioners become more aware of their bodies and how they move. For people who have back pain, such awareness can help them learn how to move without pain while gaining strength, flexibility, and the many other benefits I just mentioned. The tai chi movements and postures warm up all the joints in the body and promote the flow of chi (see Acupuncture). Other benefits may include the following:

- The practice of tai chi emphasizes correct form—no slouching or rounded shoulders, achieving a neutral spine—through consistent, routine practice, preferably every day.
- Practicing tai chi may reduce back pain, as it relieves the stress placed on the spine from poor posture.

- Tai chi involves shifting the weight from one leg to the other, flexing the joints, and extending the limbs, all of which help improve balance. Improved balance helps reduce awkward movements that can aggravate existing back pain.
- The gentle repetition of tai chi movements tones and strengthens the muscles around the spine, including the stomach and hamstring muscles, which in turn improves posture and reduces back pain.
- The deep breathing that is done along with tai chi movements helps relieve stress.

Scientific research supports the benefits patients and health-care professionals alike attribute to tai chi. One study among postmenopausal women, for example, found that tai chi training may improve bone density and neuromuscular function. Another found improved knee muscle strength and balance control among people who practiced tai chi when compared with those who did not. When it comes to reports that tai chi can improve balance and prevent falls, many studies support these claims.

Is Tai Chi for You?

Tai chi's gentle nature makes it accessible to nearly everyone. People who find some aerobic exercises to be painful or uncomfortable can greatly benefit from tai chi because it is low impact and slow moving, yet it builds strength and flexibility and improves posture. No equipment is needed, and it can be practiced just about anywhere.

I recommend taking tai chi classes rather than trying to learn it from a book or video. Only a knowledgeable instructor can accurately demonstrate and help you with the precise, fluid movements and postures of tai chi. Each motion can be modified to fit your particular ability level, and a qualified instructor can help you make those changes. Therefore, it's best to look for an instructor who has worked with back pain patients.

Tai chi sessions are typically held in small groups and last about an hour. For help locating a tai chi class near you, ask your physical therapist or local rehabilitation center.

Tai Chi: Getting Started

- Take it slow. Tai chi is a slow-moving discipline that has been likened to poetry in motion. Moving slowly and deliberately sounds easy, but it's not. Be patient; it will take some time to become accustomed to the movements.

- Practice tai chi every day. You may have class only once or twice a week, but your practice in between is important, even if it's only ten minutes a day.

- Begin every tai chi session with about five minutes of warm-up exercises.

- Breathe correctly. This integral part of tai chi can be challenging to master at first. Basically, your breathing follows your movements: open movements (arms opening wide, stepping forward) call for an "in" breath, while close movements (stepping back, drawing your arms toward your body) call for an "out" breath. Since every open movement is followed by a close movement, you should quickly find yourself breathing correctly.

- Consult your doctor before starting a tai chi program.

YOGA

Priscilla, who recently returned to work part-time at a florist shop, has become an enthusiastic advocate of yoga. "I can't tell you how much better I feel since I started yoga," she said. "My back has been bothering me for years, and except for pills, which I hate to take, nothing has helped me as much as yoga. I had epidural injections and ultrasound, which were somewhat helpful, but in the long run, yoga is the best. I never thought I'd be taking up yoga at sixty-one, but I truly believe it helped me return to work after having to quit three years ago."

Although many people associate the practice of yoga with spiritual enlightenment, it has definite physical healing benefits as well. Much depends on the type of yoga you practice, as some forms put more emphasis on strength, flexibility, posture, and balance than others. One of those types is hatha yoga, which is the most commonly practiced form in the United States. *Ha* means sun, and *tha* means moon, and thus hatha yoga is viewed as the union of opposites. This yoga form focuses on postures (asanas) and breath control, which, when combined, energize the body and mind.

Foreign Yet Familiar

It's not unusual for people to discover that some of the exercises or poses they've been given by their physical therapists or rehabilitation therapists are yoga poses. "Hey, I've done these exercises before," noted Michael, a forty-one-year-old real estate broker who reluctantly went to yoga classes to lessen his back pain at the insistence of his wife. "I never realized that my physical therapist had given me some yoga as part of my exercise routine. I guess yoga isn't as strange as I thought it was."

Yoga for Your Back

Although yoga has been found to be very effective in relieving back pain and helping prevent future episodes, not all yoga poses are recommended for people who have back conditions. Indeed, you can aggravate your existing problems if you do inappropriate poses. Therefore, it is best to do yoga under the supervision of a certified yoga instructor and/or a physical therapist or other health-care professional who is knowledgeable about the practice. Because cost may be a factor, you can attend just a few sessions with a yoga instructor to learn proper form and posture and then practice at home.

Here are three common yoga poses that may be familiar to you if you have worked with a physical therapist or taken yoga classes. These poses are often used for people who have back pain, but you should consult your doctor before you do these or any other yoga poses. Each pose should be held for five to ten seconds, depending on your comfort level, and done on a soft, supportive surface, such as an exercise mat.

- **Easy Bridge** (strengthens the abdominal, hamstring, and buttocks muscles; improves the curves in the lower back): Lie on your back and place a folded blanket under your shoulders. Bend your knees and place your feet flat on the floor. Keep your heels as close to your buttocks as is comfortable and about hip-width apart. Place your arms at your sides with palms up and keep your eyes fixed on your knees throughout the exercise. Exhale and use your abdominal muscles to press your lower back into the floor. Your pelvis should tilt. Hold this pose as you inhale. On your next exhale, press your feet firmly into the floor and slowly lift your buttocks six to eight inches off the floor (or as high as is comfortable). Continue to breathe easily, and keep your shoulders and face relaxed and your pelvis tilted. To prevent your weight from shifting, press your inner heels down firmly. Hold this raised position for five to ten seconds, then slowly return to the starting position as you exhale. Repeat the entire sequence three to five times.

- **Knee to Chest Pose** (stretches the hamstrings and opens up the lower back): Lie flat on your back on a padded surface. Slowly and gently bring one knee toward your chest. Place your hands under the knee and gently pull it toward you until you reach a comfortable position. Hold this pose for ten to fifteen seconds, then slowly return your leg to the floor. Repeat with the other leg.

- **Palm Tree** (relaxes and aligns the spine): Stand with your feet facing forward and shoulder-width apart with your weight evenly distributed. Your arms should be relaxed at your sides. Raise both arms over your head, interlock your fingers, and turn your hands so that your palms face upward. Stretch your arms upward and, at the same time, rise up on your toes. Hold this pose for five to ten seconds. If you cannot rise up on your toes without pain or if it is difficult to stay balanced, just do the over-the-head stretch. Return your arms to their original position. Repeat the exercise three to five times.

Benefits of Yoga

- Builds strength. In yoga, you are taught to hold various poses, many of which gently strengthen the muscles in the back and abdomen. This action helps you maintain proper posture and both prevents and reduces back pain.

- Stretches and relaxes. We know that stretching is very important for people who have lower back pain, and many yoga poses gently stretch the muscles necessary for back health. Yoga stretches also increase blood flow and reduce tension in constricted muscles.
- Improves balance and posture. Regular yoga practice helps align the spine and strengthens both sides of the body equally, which contribute to improved balance and a neutral spine.
- Enhances body awareness. As you become more aware of your body, you can more easily recognize its strengths and limitations, which then helps you determine which movements can be done safely and which ones should be avoided.
- Reduces stress. Yoga has long been associated with stress reduction and allowing people to enter a mental state of calm, positive thinking, and balance.
- Modifies easily. Many yoga poses are suitable for people who have chronic lower back pain, but simple modifications can always be made if you have special needs or have considerable pain. Therefore, I strongly suggest you work with a yoga instructor who is knowledgeable about back pain and how to modify yoga movements or make simple adjustments, such as placing a pillow or folded towel under the knees to reduce strain on the lower back.

Is Yoga for You?

Research shows that yoga is proving to be helpful for many people who suffer with back pain. At the West Virginia University School of Medicine, for example, investigators found that patients who participated in a sixteen-week program of Iyengar yoga (an intense yoga form that concentrates on strength and flexibility) had significant reductions in pain intensity, disability, and medication use immediately following and three months after the study ended. In another study, this one of hatha yoga, investigators found that patients who participated in one-hour sessions twice weekly for six weeks had improved balance and flexibility and reduced disability and depression.

In addition to hatha and Iyengar yoga, there are many other types from which to choose. Kripalu, for example, focuses on developing your physical, emotional, and spiritual states through exercises (asanas), breathing, and meditation. Kundalini yoga is often regarded as a more spiritually based form that pairs deep, rhythmic breathing with movement. Regardless of the yoga form you choose, you should always consult your doctor or physical therapist before you begin to practice yoga, and look for an instructor who has worked with people who have back pain. You can consult the resources section for the names of professional organizations that can provide additional information and referrals.

BODY AIDS

"Sure, my back hurts all the time," said Roger, a forty-eight-year-old plumber. "But I have my own business and a family to support, and I can't afford to be out of work. So I found some things that make my life a little less painful, and they really help." Because Roger spends a great deal of time driving his truck from job to job, he found he needed some lower back support, so he bought a lumbar roll for the front seat. He was also having a great deal of trouble sleeping, so he researched various types of mattresses until he found one that allows him to sleep well.

The right body aid can make a big difference in your level of pain or discomfort, the amount of sleep you get, your job productivity, and your mood. Appropriate chairs, mattresses, or accessories may make a significant difference in your quality of life, whether it's at home, in the office, in your car, or when you travel. I recommend that my patients evaluate their lifestyle and discuss with their doctor or physical therapist how a body aid may provide them with much-needed or additional comfort and/or support for their back and overall health. Let's look at some of these basic body aids.

Please Be Seated

It's a common misconception: many people believe that when they sit down, they are relaxing and taking stress off their back. What actually happens is that the entire upper body's weight is transferred onto the thighs and buttocks, and pressure on the intervertebral discs increases to three times more than it is when you are standing. As you likely already know, sitting can be very uncomfortable, even impossible, if you have back pain. If you sit incorrectly, especially without back support, it can lead to poor posture, aggravate your back pain, and also result in leg, neck, and/or abdominal pain.

About 70 percent of America's workforce sits on the job. If you add to that the time spent commuting to work, watching television, and interacting with a personal computer, you can see that Americans tend to sit a lot. Having a chair that supports or promotes a healthy back can be very important if your job and/or lifestyle requires that you sit for extended periods. One option is an ergonomic office chair, which can help reduce back pain and fatigue, improve blood flow, and increase productivity. Here's what to look for.

- **Seat.** Select a chair with a cushion that is composed of spring coils or dense padding. You want to avoid a cushion that will compress over time and ultimately cause imbalance and back fatigue. The seat should be at least one inch wider than your hips and thighs on both sides, and the front of the seat should slope down slightly to allow your knees to be lower than your hips. The space between the back of your knees and the front edge of the seat should be about the size of your fist to help reduce pressure on the back of your thighs. If possible, also look for a chair that has a sliding mechanism that allows you to adjust the distance between the seat and the backrest.
- **Backrest.** The main function of the backrest is to offer support to the lumbar spine. The backrest should be either small enough to fit into the small of your back or curved to offer support. Many chairs have a knob on the side of the chair that allows you to adjust the backrest.
- **Armrests.** Not everyone likes armrests, and often they can be distracting. If you want or need armrests, however, look for ones that are adjustable and that are at least 2 inches wide to adequately support your arms.
- **Seat Height.** Your chair needs to be at a height that allows you to rest your feet properly on the floor while your upper body is correctly aligned with your desk, computer, or other work area. "Properly" means your feet should be flat on the floor and your knees should be slightly lower than your hips. Chairs typically can be ad-

justed using either a hydraulic or pneumatic adjustment mechanism; the latter allows you to adjust the seat height while you are sitting on the chair.

- **Footrest.** Most people don't need a footrest, but if you use one, your knees should still be lower than your hips.

SITTING PRETTY

- Don't just sit there—move. A healthy body is not designed to stay in one position for more than about twenty minutes. When you sit too long, you slowly stretch the elasticity out of your tissues, which allows stress to accumulate in your muscles and cause pain. Therefore, if possible, stand up and stretch every twenty minutes or so. You don't need to get out of your chair to move: stretch your arms up over your head, extend each leg individually and rotate your ankles, and lift each leg separately from the seat.

- Sit straight with your shoulders and back against the backrest.

- If you have armrests, allow your elbows and lower arms to rest on them lightly. Do not use the armrests to slouch.

- Keep your shoulders relaxed and slightly dropped if you are using a keyboard.

- Maintain a healthy, neutral position: make sure your hips are slightly higher than your knees, keep your back supported, equally distribute your weight on the seat cushion, and keep two to four inches of space between the back of your knees and the edge of the chair.

Back and Neck Supports

This is a broad category that includes supports marketed as pillows, wedges, rolls, and cushions, all designed to help support the back and/or parts of the body that have an impact on the back and neck. Back supports, for example, help support your weight and prevent your spine from sinking into cushions that are too soft. They can be used in your car, at home on soft chairs and sofas, and with inadequate office chairs. Lumbar rolls are a type of back support popular with people who drive a lot and who need additional support behind their lower spine. Another item is a cushion support seat, which typically adjusts your weight to relieve pressure points and helps prevent lower back pain. Such cushions are light and portable and so can be taken anywhere, such as sporting events, restaurants, and other places that may have chairs you will find uncomfortable.

Using such supports is a personal choice. Some patients take their cushion support seats or special lumbar rolls or pillows with them wherever they go. Others say they don't need these items. Consult your doctor or physical therapist about supports and whether he or she thinks you may benefit from any of them. Then try them out: purchase items only from companies or stores that will allow you to return them within a reasonable amount of time if they do not work for you. There are dozens of outlets for support items; talk to your physician or physical therapist, or check out the Internet for sources.

Choosing a Mattress

Considering that we spend approximately one-third of our lives sleeping—or trying to sleep—finding the right mattress is important. If you have chronic low back pain, finding that mattress is an even more critical matter. It's a mixed blessing that there are so many different mattresses on the market from which to choose. But variety is what you want, because no single mattress is best for everyone who has low back pain. With that in mind, here are some guidelines for choosing a mattress for comfort and support.

- Although many doctors have traditionally recommended that their patients who have back pain sleep on a firm mattress, a recent study published in the prestigious medical journal *The Lancet* reported that patients who slept on a medium-firm mattress were more likely to experience reduced back pain in bed, less pain when they got out of bed, and less back pain related to disability than patients who slept on a firm mattress. The study, which involved 313 adults, found that a medium-firm mattress provided a better balance between lower back comfort and lower back support than did a firm mattress. That's not to say everyone preferred the medium-firm mattress over a firm one, which means it is still a matter of personal preference.
- The number and placement of coils in the mattress determine the amount of support the mattress provides, while the amount of padding determines the comfort level. The wire comes in different thicknesses: a lower gauge number means a thicker, stiffer wire and thus a firmer mattress. Some people find that a firm mattress with some added padding works best for them. Mattresses that have more coils and thicker padding are usually higher in quality and more expensive, but a high price tag is no guarantee that a mattress offers superior support or comfort.

- If you have an old mattress that sags, it's probably time to get a new one. You can put boards under the mattress, but this is a quick fix only and is ultimately unsatisfying.
- Don't be fooled by claims that a mattress is "orthopedic" or "approved by doctors." You are the ultimate expert when it comes to finding a comfortable mattress.
- If possible, test a mattress before you buy it. Unfortunately, testing a mattress in a showroom doesn't give you enough time or information to make a decision. If you have a family member or friend who has a mattress brand you are considering, perhaps you can sleep on it for a night or two. You can also check with hotels to see what types of mattresses they have.
- If you can't test a mattress adequately before you buy it, the next best thing is to purchase your mattress from a store that will allow you to return it within a reasonable amount of time (at least ten days, preferably thirty) if you are not satisfied with the comfort or quality of sleep.
- The mattress foundation or box spring also affects comfort and sleep quality. Wooden frames may make your mattress feel harder than a frame that has springs. According to the Better Sleep Council, it is best to purchase a foundation and mattress as a set because it maximizes the life of the mattress.
- Some people prefer a mattress composed of memory foam, a general term for a material that automatically adjusts to a person's body weight and temperature. Memory foam can eliminate uncomfortable pressure points and thus relieve pains and aches that can make it difficult for you to sleep.
- Once you find the right mattress, take care of it. Rotate it 180 degrees and flip it lengthwise every six months.

(Note: Do not attempt this on your own. Ask someone to do it for you!)

IN CONCLUSION . . .

Body therapies and body aids should be on your "check it out" list for your back pain treatment and maintenance plan. Four of the six body therapies discussed in this chapter—massage, Pilates, tai chi, and yoga—are approaches you can learn and do at home (with your doctor's approval). Acupuncture and chiropractic require professionals, who are easily accessible in most cities in the United States today. All of the body therapies discussed are excellent integrative approaches that can complement other therapies you may be using, including medication and a home exercise program. If you haven't tried any of these therapies, I encourage you to add one or more of them, if appropriate, to your life.

Chapter 5

Step 3: Minding Your Back

For a few moments, let's switch our focus away from the body and turn to the mind and what psychology can contribute to the treatment of chronic pain. Actually, diverting our attention in this way is not so easy to do because there is such an intimate relationship between body and mind. This relationship is definitely to our advantage, as you'll discover in this chapter, in which I talk about how you can enjoy the benefits of several psychology-based mind-body techniques that are effective in the management of chronic back pain. These natural, noninvasive approaches can provide significant relief and be welcome complements to other remedies you may be using, including an exercise program. Psychologist Raymond Hanlon, of the University of Pittsburgh Medical Center Pain Medicine Program, suggests that mind-body, psychology-based approaches to chronic pain management are not only alternatives to standard medical therapy but also an essential part of integrated, multidisciplinary treatment for chronic pain. In fact, patients frequently find that one or more of the therapies that I discuss in this chapter, along with routine exercise and use of appropriate medical approaches, are all they need to successfully manage their chronic back pain.

In this chapter, I discuss ways you can "use your head" to handle chronic pain and also deal with the depression that often accompanies it. Of the many different mind-body approaches, I have chosen those whose effectiveness is supported by research as well as the reports of many satisfied patients who have benefited from them. Included in our discussion are biofeedback, breathing therapy, cognitive-behavioral therapy, self-hypnosis, meditation, and visualization/guided imagery. I offer some guidelines on how you can incorporate these techniques into your life and/or provide resources for locating practitioners, and note which painful conditions respond to each therapy. Several patients share their experiences with different approaches.

ENTERING THE MIND-BODY EXPERIENCE

As it's become increasingly evident that the mainstays of conventional medicine—drugs and/or invasive procedures, including surgery—are often far from ideal when it comes to preventing and treating chronic low back pain, many patients are looking for effective, safe options. I'm happy to say that there are numerous such alternatives available and that I have known many patients who have benefited from them. Many people have come to me after having spent years going to doctors who never suggested or even mentioned any of the mind-body techniques, even though there is growing scientific proof and certainly much anecdotal evidence to support the use of a significant number of them.

That being said, I want to emphasize that the options discussed in this chapter should be viewed as complementary to whatever treatment approaches you are already using or are in the process of selecting. Raymond Hanlon emphasizes that you can increase the benefits achievable from mind-body techniques when these approaches are learned and utilized as part of a multidisciplinary treatment plan. Unfortunately, chronic pain management clinics that offer such programs are often limited to large medical centers, and thus these programs are not widely accessible. However, patients who do not take part in these programs for whatever reason can still seek help from individual practitioners who can provide needed services and help them incorporate information they glean from this book.

Do not, for example, abruptly stop taking the anti-inflammatory drug you've used daily for six months when you first try visualization. Wait until you begin to reap the benefits of this mind-body technique. That's not to say that you can't enjoy sufficient pain relief using mind-body therapies alone, as indeed many people do. *Mind-body therapies can be every bit as powerful as medication—but without the side effects*—so they should be entered into with that thought in mind.

Benefits of Deep Relaxation

One reason these techniques are so powerful, when done correctly, is that they help you to reach a state of deep relaxation—a health-enhancing state. A sad truth is that *many people don't know how to truly relax.* Their idea of relaxation is to have a cocktail or two after work, drink a cup of coffee and smoke a cigarette, or indulge in a pint of double chocolate chip ice cream. Unfortunately, some people turn to sleeping pills or other sedatives to help them "relax." Although all of these substances may help you *feel* relaxed temporarily, they are ultimately harmful to your physical and psychological health and in the long run create more stress in your life.

Mind-body therapies can take you to a truly deep, relaxed state. Deep relaxation has a direct impact on the autonomic nervous system, helping it rid the body of tension, anxiety, and stress. It helps quiet the mind, which in turn reduces activity in the sympathetic nervous system and stimulates the parasympathetic system. This combination relaxes your muscles, and when muscles relax, they lengthen, which promotes blood flow and results in a reduction in inflammation and swelling. Improved blood flow also delivers more nutrition and oxygen to your muscles while removing toxins. In short, deep relaxation promotes healing and relieves pain essentially by reducing the brain's awareness of pain signals. This concept is based on the medical community's widely accepted conceptualization of the human experience of pain.

Of course, there are other advantages associated with mind-body approaches, including their relatively low or no cost and the sense of personal control they can give you. As one patient said, "Once I learned self-hypnosis, I had the freedom to deal with my pain on my terms. I now know that I can tap into what I've learned at any time and that I'll soon feel better. It isn't perfect, but neither were the pills I was depending on, and I hated the side effects." Practicing relaxation techniques also leaves you feeling physically energized and mentally more aware.

I encourage you, as I encourage my patients, to approach the techniques in this chapter with an open mind and with the view that they are yet more ways to overcome the pain and put you in control.

BIOFEEDBACK

Biofeedback is a two-pronged technique: it's a type of behavior conditioning and a relaxation technique combined. The basic goal of biofeedback is to help you control certain physiological functions, such as body temperature, heart rate, breathing rate, brain wave activity, and muscle tension, as a means of reducing pain and decreasing the effects of stress. When it comes to back pain, biofeedback has been used to measure the electrical activity of muscles in the back and to train patients to reduce tension and muscle activity associated with their pain. Therefore, biofeedback can be an effective approach for chronic low back pain associated with myofascial pain, fibromyalgia, strains, and spasm.

Unlike the other mind-body techniques discussed in this chapter, biofeedback requires the use of equipment, at least initially, until you learn how to control certain body functions on your own. With practice, however, you will be able to achieve your goals without the monitoring devices, which means you will then be able to reap the relaxation and tension-reduction benefits of the biofeedback technique wherever you are.

How It Works

Biofeedback sessions are usually conducted in a quiet room where you can make yourself comfortable in a chair or by lying down. The sessions are facilitated by a biofeedback therapist, who teaches you various relaxation techniques, such as visualization, deep breathing, and progressive relaxation, to help you relax and make biofeedback work for you. The type of biofeedback typically used for back pain is electromyographic (EMG) biofeedback, in which electrodes (or sensors) are placed on your skin over the muscles to be monitored. For low back pain, electrodes are often placed in the lumbar region, although they may be placed in other areas as well (e.g., the shoulder muscles, which many people hunch when they are stressed).

When the electrodes detect tension in a muscle, the computerized monitoring device, which is hooked up to the electrodes, emits a signal, such as a beep or a colored light on a monitor. Over time, you recognize how it feels when your muscles are tense and how to know when the tension is beginning to build. You can then use whatever relaxation techniques you have learned to control or stop the tension before it goes any further and causes pain.

Loreen's Story

Loreen had been trying to cope with low back pain for more than three years. She remembered first feeling the pain when she went waterskiing for her thirty-third birthday. A bad fall left more than her ego bruised, and she experienced flares of moderately severe pain every few months, with mild to moderate pain in between, ever since then. A recent promotion at work meant she had to be on her feet more than in the past, and she was looking for a way to cope with what she knew would be a chronically painful experience. She was already taking anti-inflammatory drugs as needed but wanted to wean herself off them if she could. A friend suggested she try biofeedback, but first she wanted some advice.

At this point, Loreen came to see me for the first time. After a thorough examination and history, I recommended she work with a physical therapist to develop an exercise program. She agreed but also wanted to know more about biofeedback. After we talked, I referred her to a pain management clinic in her area that offered biofeedback.

At the clinic, the therapist asked Loreen whether she had ever tried any relaxation techniques, such as visualization or self-hypnosis. Although she had not, she expressed an interest in visualization and guided imagery, so the therapist placed the electrodes on Loreen's lumbar region and then explained how these therapies work (see Visualization and Guided Imagery later in this chapter). Before they tried any visualization or guided imagery, however, the therapist asked Loreen to concentrate on relaxing her muscles and releasing the tension in her back and shoulders. Although Loreen said she was "trying to relax," the nearly steady beep of the monitor told a different story. "Remember that sound," said the therapist. "Now you're going to learn how to make it go away."

The therapist then led Loreen through a guided imagery session, which focused on ideas Loreen gave her about how much she enjoyed visiting her family's cabin and lake in Vermont. She then encouraged Loreen to work on visualization and guided imagery that incorporated all the sights, sounds, tastes, textures, and smells from her favorite place in Vermont and to use them during her biofeedback sessions and when she practiced at home.

After just two more sessions, Loreen was able to noticeably reduce the beeps coming from the monitor. "I realized that there were some sights and smells I would bring to mind that were more powerful than others," said Loreen. "There's a grove of pine trees near the cabin that smells heavenly in the fall, and I feel almost giddy when I stand among them. Now I find I can conjure up that smell and that image and it makes me relax more than some other images do. I never realized how powerful this could be!"

After several weeks of twice-weekly sessions, Loreen learned to identify the tension in her back and how to release it with guided imagery. She weaned herself off the monitoring device and, to her surprise, many of her anti-inflammatory drugs as well, although she occasionally turns to them "to take the edge off the pain." She says she's "pretty good" about doing her stretching and strength exercises at home, and says that her biofeedback experience helps her a lot with pain management, especially on the job.

Is Biofeedback for You?

Not all studies of biofeedback used specifically for treatment of back pain have shown the technique to be beneficial. However, there is evidence of its usefulness in relieving specific areas of tension, so if muscle tension is contributing in specific ways to your chronic back pain, then biofeedback may help you. It is painless, has no side effects, and once learned, can be done just about anywhere and at any time.

But biofeedback isn't for everyone. It requires a time commitment to learn the technique, which typically takes several sessions per week for two to three weeks. You also need to be willing to learn different relaxation methods to alter the feedback, such as meditation, visualization, or self-hypnosis, as these relaxation techniques are what actually result in a reduction in muscle tension and pain. The biofeedback equipment is simply a tool that provides you with cues that can help you get the most benefit from your relaxation efforts. To help you with these tasks, you will need to work with a biofeedback specialist and/or a facility that offers biofeedback. Fortunately, biofeedback has gained considerable acceptance among medical professionals as a pain management approach, and so it is now part of the program in a growing number of pain clinics, integrative medicine facilities, and physical therapy offices.

Raymond Hanlon suggests that many individuals who have

long-standing chronic back pain may also have tension throughout the body. In such cases, biofeedback may be less effective than more generalized relaxation techniques, such as breathing or progressive muscle relaxation, in reducing both back pain and the widespread tension.

Biofeedback should be viewed as a complementary treatment, one to be used along with other approaches, including a home exercise program. It usually takes several weeks of training before you can gain the amount of control that will significantly reduce your pain. Basically, if you are highly motivated and a little patient, you will likely succeed and have an effective tool forever at your disposal.

BREATHING THERAPY

When I tell patients that something as simple as breathing properly can help relieve their chronic back pain, I get skeptical looks, but they're usually also curious. The secret, I explain, is learning to breathe *properly* during times of stress, tension, and pain. Infants, because they have not yet developed responses to psychosocial stressors, have it right: they breathe from the diaphragm, which causes the belly to rise and fall. Adults, when in stressful situations, breathe from the chest and take shallow breaths as a natural learned response to stress, such as pain. Learning to breathe from the diaphragm in these situations reduces tension and perceived stress.

When people are taught how to breathe correctly, several things happen. One benefit is that more oxygen gets into the bloodstream, which carries it to the muscles in the back, which in turn promotes strengthening and healing. Another plus is that proper breathing is more efficient and relaxed, which has a soothing effect on the brain and nervous system, which in turn reduces overall tension in the body and the perception of pain. A third advantage of proper breathing is that it improves body awareness.

Why is improved body awareness important in pain relief? Studies show that people with chronic back pain have difficulty with proprioception, which is sometimes referred to as the sixth sense. Proprioception gives you a sense of awareness of where your body or a part of your body is in space; it is a sensory feedback process by which the body immediately alters muscle contractions in response to information as it comes in from external sources. Lumbar disc herniation at L4 and/or L5, for example, can cause loss of proprioception in one or both legs, which can cause significant problems.

For example, imagine you are walking across a room covered with thick carpet and you unexpectedly step down on a marble that is hidden in the rug. The muscles in your feet and legs adjust immediately to the new sensory information they receive. This new information is sensed by proprioceptors, which send the information to your brain, and your muscles make adjustments, which helps you keep your balance. Proprioception helps with posture and motor control as well. If your proprioception is compromised, you risk falling and injuring yourself.

A recent study from Germany notes that breathing therapy is effective because it enhances proprioception, which is deficient in patients who have chronic back pain. It's uncertain whether this is true, but other studies support the effectiveness of breathing therapy in relieving pain in patients with chronic back pain. At the University of California, San Francisco, for example, breathing therapy was compared with physical therapy in a controlled trial that lasted six to eight weeks. The patients participated in twelve sessions of either breathing or physical therapy, and at the end of the study, both groups reported a similar improvement in pain. Patients in the breathing therapy group also showed improved coping skills and had gained a new perspective on the effect stress has on the body.

Breathing for Back Pain Relief

Breathing therapy involves more than simply breathing in and out; it is also part meditation, part movement therapy. In fact, you will notice that in our discussions of meditation, tai chi, and yoga, for example, breathing is an integral part of each practice. The several different breathing methods we discuss here can help reduce back pain and restore balance to the entire body, but they can also be used along with these other therapies. You may want to refer back to this section for breathing tips when you are reading the other sections.

Here are four short breathing techniques and one longer one that patients find to be helpful in alleviating pain. Breathing exercises are especially popular to use with biofeedback and self-hypnosis and to help people fall asleep.

- **Basic Deep Breathing.** Lie down on your back with your knees bent, or sit in a chair, whichever is more comfortable for your back. Place your open palms on your abdomen and rib cage so you can feel them move as you breathe. Take a deep breath through your nose and send the breath deep into your abdomen. As you do, you should feel your belly rise. Your diaphragm and upper lungs should expand as well. Hold that breath for a few seconds, then slowly release it through your mouth. Slowly repeat this cycle several times, always being conscious of sending your breath into your abdomen, diaphragm, and lungs. Once you feel comfortable with this exercise, try the next breathing technique, hatha breathing.

- **Hatha Breathing.** While in your comfortable position, take one hand and place it on a spot three finger-widths below your navel. This spot is one of the acupressure points, known as Conception Vessel 6, and is regarded as a high energy site. Concentrate on this spot as you take a deep breath and send the air into your belly. Feel your lower abdomen rise and fall as you breathe slowly in and out. Continue to focus on your breathing for several minutes. This breathing exercise helps strengthen the lower back.
- **Breath Meditation.** This is an example of combining two approaches. Details can be found under Meditation later in this chapter.
- **Breath Visualization.** An exercise in which you visualize your breath as a healing substance can be very powerful (see Visualization and Guided Imagery later in this chapter). This is a popular approach to use with biofeedback and when you find it difficult to sleep.

Progressive Breathing

This breathing exercise can help relax your back and calm your mind and nervous system. Progressive breathing takes more practice than the previous breathing exercises, so be patient. Allow yourself ten to fifteen minutes to complete each session.

1. Lie down on your back with your knees bent. If you need to place pillows under your hips, neck, or knees to feel more comfortable, do so.
2. Close your eyes and slowly inhale a deep, full breath. Imagine that you can feel the air reach into your abdomen. Keep inhaling until your abdomen is completely

expanded and then, without pausing, slowly exhale until it is completely empty.

3. Take another deep breath and fully expand your abdomen. Then notice the air as it enters your chest and fully expands your rib cage.

4. Once your abdomen and chest are fully expanded, slowly exhale by first emptying your chest and rib cage and then your abdomen. Try to keep the movement of air smooth and even; do not strain. Practice breathing this way (into your abdomen and chest) for several minutes until you feel comfortable.

5. Take a deep breath that fills your abdomen, chest, and rib cage, and then focus your attention on your shoulders. Notice how they rise slightly as you breathe deeply.

6. When you have inhaled completely, relax and release your breath slowly through your mouth, allowing it to leave first from your shoulders, then your chest and rib cage, then your abdomen. Empty your breath completely from each of these body areas before you move on to the next one.

7. Repeat steps five and six for several minutes.

8. Return to your normal breathing pattern. Notice how your back feels and how you feel overall.

Is Breathing Therapy for You?

Quite simply, why not? Once relaxation breathing techniques are learned, they do not require professional help or equipment; they can be done just about anywhere and at any time, there are no side effects, and they're free. The breathing techniques discussed here and those you can find elsewhere (see Suggested Reading) can be used in conjunction with meditation, self-hypnosis, visualization and guided imagery, yoga, and various other treatment options. I encourage you to make breathing therapy a part of your daily routine and see if it makes a positive difference. What do you have to lose, except pain?

COGNITIVE-BEHAVIORAL THERAPY

Cognitive-behavioral therapy is based on scientific research that suggests that your thoughts—not external events, circumstances, or other people—influence your feelings and behaviors. You have the power to change the way you think, act, and feel about a specific situation, even if you have no control over the situation you are in. Thus, positive change can occur when you learn to think constructively, and that applies to how you think about, feel and act toward, and live with your chronic pain.

Cognitive-behavioral therapy is a standard approach used in multidisciplinary chronic pain treatment programs and clinics. Participating in this type of therapy to help you deal with chronic pain, as many people do, does not mean your pain isn't real or that you have a psychological problem. It means that you are willing to utilize a powerful treatment to help you modify the thoughts, attitudes, feelings, and behaviors that can contribute to the stress, tension, and depression caused by pain.

Cognitive-Behavioral Therapy: Does It Work?

In 1995, a twelve-member panel convened by the National Institutes of Health at the NIH Technology Assessment Conference on the Integration of Behavioral and Relaxation Approaches into the Treatment of Chronic Pain and Insomnia stated that cognitive-behavioral techniques are effective in alleviating chronic pain, especially low back pain and arthritis. Indeed, many studies support this recommendation.

In a 1988 study, for example, researchers found that cognitive-behavioral therapy was useful in significantly decreasing physical and psychosocial disability in patients with chronic low back pain when compared with a control group, even up to twelve months after treatment ended. Another study, this one in England in 1995, compared the effectiveness of eight sessions of cognitive-behavioral therapy or biofeedback with controls in forty-four patients who had chronic low back pain. Treated patients reported significant improvement in pain, depression, beliefs about pain, and disability compared with control patients. Six months later, patients in both of the treatment groups still had improvement in the first three areas, and also improved in how they used their active coping skills. Two more recent review studies (2000 and 2005) conducted by the same team at the Institute for Research in Extramural Medicine found that cognitive-behavioral therapy is effective for chronic low back pain and has a positive effect on pain intensity.

What to Expect from Cognitive-Behavioral Therapy

Cognitive-behavioral therapy for pain management is usually offered weekly in small group sessions led by a psychiatrist, psychologist, or behavioral health professional specifically trained in cognitive-behavior therapy. If you decide to consult a psychotherapist trained in cognitive-behavioral therapy, expect to learn how your perception and behavior can affect how you experience pain, and that when you modify disturbed thoughts, you can play a role in modifying your pain. You will be taught coping skills—ways to change your perception of pain, plus ways to adapt your behavior—and relaxation exercises, such as progressive relaxation exercises, visualization, distraction techniques, and meditation. The therapist will introduce you to cognitive restructuring—helping you identify and challenge any overly negative pain-related thoughts you have and showing you how to replace them with coping thoughts and behaviors.

Cognitive-behavioral therapy is also effective in either warding off depression or learning how to manage it head on. As we discussed in chapter 1, I believe it is important to identify and treat depression as part of an effective management plan for chronic low back pain.

ShariAnn's Story

ShariAnn is a forty-eight-year-old software developer who has a long history of low back pain and fibromyalgia, both of which she has managed with NSAIDs, periodic massage, and mild opioids, when necessary, for the past fifteen years. She often has trouble sleeping, despite buying what she calls her "million-dollar mattress," and she has made arrangements at work to leave early or to work at home about half the time because she needs to rest during the day.

One of her co-workers was driving too fast through the parking lot one afternoon and crashed into ShariAnn's car as she sat waiting for another co-worker to back out of a parking spot. The impact was enough to send ShariAnn's back into spasms, and she was out of work for three weeks, and then was able to return only part-time because of the pain. After the accident, ShariAnn went to her doctor, who recommended trigger-point therapy as a prelude to an exercise program developed by a physical therapist that included McKenzie Method exercises and gentle stretching.

Immediately after the accident, ShariAnn became very angry with the co-worker who had hit her, Renee, and resented that Renee hadn't suffered even a scratch from the incident. ShariAnn was also very afraid she would be laid off because she couldn't work as much as she had before the accident, and she was depressed because her back pain was now much worse than it had been in years. ShariAnn's doctor was concerned about her negative mood and suggested she see a psychotherapist for cognitive-behavioral therapy. She protested, but her husband persuaded her to give it a try.

The therapist worked with ShariAnn on how to think differently about the accident and her anger toward Renee and helped her realize that her anger was unproductive and, worse, causing her physical stress and pain. "I realized I could either choose to be miserable and blame Renee for my pain and feel sorry for myself—essentially let the situation control me—or I could take back control of my life," said ShariAnn. She decided to learn meditation and visualization and began to practice them daily to help her with painful flares and when she had difficulty sleeping. The therapist also gave her an assignment: to read something inspirational every day for at least fifteen minutes, whether it was spiritual, religious, or motivational self-help in nature, and to meditate on what she read.

After a month of therapy, ShariAnn decided to meet with her co-worker face-to-face for the first time since the accident. "My meditation and visualization were going well, and I felt I had some control over my life again," she said. "But something was unfinished, and I knew it was time for me to rethink my anger. My therapist kept saying, 'If something isn't working, change it.'

Well, my anger toward Renee wasn't working, so I had to make a change." ShariAnn contacted Renee and asked if they could meet for coffee at a café. At the end of their two-hour meeting, they were giving each other a hug.

"Renee and I probably won't become best friends," says ShariAnn, "but we talked and discovered we had a lot in common: we're both moms, our kids go to the same schools, and we find it hard to juggle a full-time job along with everything else we need to do. I know she's terribly sorry about the accident. And believe it or not, I actually feel better physically now that I've talked to Renee."

Is Cognitive-Behavioral Therapy for You?

Cognitive-behavioral therapy requires commitment on your part, as you'll need to practice monitoring and modifying your thoughts, practice relaxation techniques, be more aware of your feelings and how you react to situations, and be willing to change behaviors, negative thoughts, and feelings. Patients who accept the challenge usually find cognitive-behavioral therapy to be effective and rewarding and that the skills and lessons they learn can be used in various situations throughout their lives.

If you need help locating a cognitive-behavioral therapist, you can consult your physician or local mental health facilities, or you can contact the National Association of Cognitive-Behavioral Therapists (see the resources section).

SELF-HYPNOSIS

"If you told me a year ago I would be practicing self-hypnosis to manage my back pain, I would have told you you're crazy," said Larry, a thirty-nine-year-old truck driver. "But I drive across country and I can't rely on drugs to control my back pain. I've got lumbar support in my rig, a memory-foam mattress in the back, and now I've got self-hypnosis to get me through the tough times."

Larry is just one of many people with chronic low back pain who have found relief using self-hypnosis. At one time largely ignored by conventional medicine, hypnosis has gained acceptance by many mainstream practitioners as they come to recognize how powerful it can be in certain situations, such as managing, reducing, and coping with chronic pain.

Hypnosis is a state of awareness, concentration, and focused attention in which individuals have an increased ability to respond to suggestions. Self-hypnosis is a method that allows you to train your mind and body to make desired changes in your life. Despite what many people believe, when you are in a hypnotic state, you do not lose control. In fact, self-hypnosis is a position of control: you voluntarily enter a state of deep relaxation, separate yourself from the issue you want to remedy (back pain, for example), and accept suggestions that will help you gain the upper hand over your situation. Self-hypnosis is only truly successful if you learn to master, or control, the process.

I am focusing on self-hypnosis because it is more practical and inexpensive than returning again and again to a hypnotherapist for one-on-one sessions. (If you prefer this approach, however, it is effective.) Once you master self-hypnosis, which you can do with the help of a professional hypnotherapist in a few sessions, you will be able to place yourself in a hypnotic state, plant positive suggestions, and then leave the hypnotic state.

How Self-Hypnosis Works

If you have ever been so engrossed in a project or a good book that you lost all track of time or were unaware of what was going on around you, then you've been in a hypnotic or trancelike state. The type of hypnotic state associated with self-hypnosis is similar, but a bit deeper.

In self-hypnosis, a trancelike state has two distinct stages. Stage one is a superficial trance in which you are very aware of your surroundings, and you will remember the entire event, unless you've been given other instructions. The trance is very light in this stage, and although you may accept suggestions, you may not act on them. A map of your brain waves would show many more beta waves (those present during a normal awake state) than alpha waves.

In stage two, or the alpha phase, the number of alpha waves increases. Alpha waves are slower than beta waves and are accompanied by a reduced heart rate, lower blood pressure, and slowed respiration. The alpha phase is the stage during which you are most open to suggestions.

Researchers have studied the brain's cerebral cortex during hypnosis and found reduced activity in the left hemisphere and increased activity in the right. Scientists believe the left hemisphere of the cortex is the center of logic and reason, while the right hemisphere controls creativity and imagination. Thus, a reduction in left-hemisphere activity supports the idea that hypnosis suppresses the conscious mind, while an increase in right-hemisphere activity supports the idea that the creative subconscious takes over. This is merely a hypothesis for the moment, but one that some experts believe holds promise.

What the Experts Say

Hypnosis has gained the approval of the National Institutes of Health (NIH). In 1995, the NIH Office of Complementary and Alternative Medicine researchers taught self-hypnosis to people who had chronic back pain. With regular practice, the patients reduced their pain by 80 percent and also reported getting a better night's sleep and being less depressed. In that same year, the NIH recommended that hypnosis be considered a part of the medical protocol for chronic pain and that insurance companies reimburse patients for this treatment.

In 1998 at Virginia Polytechnic Institute and State University, Dr. Helen Crawford and her fellow investigators found that after three hypnotic sessions, patients with chronic low back pain reported pain reduction, improved sleep quality, and increased psychological well-being. Several years later, Dr. Crawford and her research team completed a study that showed that highly hypnotizable, healthy adults have a significantly larger rostrum, an area of the brain associated with attention and the transfer of information, than people who are not highly hypnotizable, and that the highly hypnotizable individuals were better able to eliminate pain perception. Studies like these support the claims that hypnosis is a scientifically viable therapeutic approach.

Is Self-Hypnosis for You?

According to Brian M. Alman, Ph.D., a clinical psychologist and author of *Self-Hypnosis: The Complete Manual for Health and Self-Change*, relief from chronic pain can be achieved after just a few sessions in which you learn how to alter the way you feel pain. Drs. Ronald Melzack and Patrick D. Wall, who are well known for their pioneering work with pain, note that self-hypnosis allows you to separate your thoughts from or turn off the area of your body that is painful by using one or more techniques, such as progressive relaxation, guided imagery, music, and breathing therapy, among others. The hypnotherapist you work with will help you decide which methods work best for you.

When you are learning hypnosis from a professional, I recommend you tape your sessions so you can use the tapes at home. Or, if you prefer, you can purchase and listen to self-help tapes that are designed to deal with chronic pain management (see the suggested reading and videos/DVDs section).

To help you feel more comfortable about self-hypnosis, here's an idea of what you can expect.

- You should be in a quiet, comfortable setting where you won't be disturbed for the length of the session, typically thirty to forty-five minutes. During your first few sessions, it may take you up to fifteen minutes to reach a fully hypnotic state and begin to focus on your goals. With practice, however, you will become much more adept at the process, and it may take only ten minutes to complete the entire session.

- You may sit or lie down, depending on your level of pain.

- Practiced, controlled breathing is the usual way to relax and clear your mind so you can more easily enter a hypnotic state. You can refer back to the Breathing Therapy section for more information on this.

- Once you have taken several deep breaths and feel comfortable, fix your eyes on an object or spot that is in front of you and above your line of vision. It can be a picture on the wall, a candle flame, a design in the wall-paper, or a crack in the window. Keep your attention focused on the spot you've chosen and continue to breathe gently, deeply, and slowly. Your hypnotherapist will prompt you with suggestions such as, "With every breath you take, you grow more and more relaxed. The more you relax, the better you feel." You may suggest other phrases that work better for you. The hypnotherapist will also offer suggestions for closing your eyes: "Your eyes feel heavy. With every breath, your eyes grow heavier and heavier."

• Most people close their eyes once they are in a hypnotic state because it helps them stay focused. However, if you prefer to keep your eyes open, you can.

• Once you are in a deeply relaxed state—in your subconscious—the therapist will introduce a post-hypnotic suggestion that you will respond to once you return to a fully conscious state. For example, a suggestion might be "When you begin to feel tense or anxious, do deep breathing exercises" or "When you begin to feel increased pain in your lower back, imagine the pain leaves your body through your fingertips and escapes into the atmosphere." The suggestions may include a prompt to do something you have found to be very relaxing or to focus on an image you've found helpful during a guided imagery session. You can get suggestions from your hypnotherapist or from self-hypnosis tapes.

MEDITATION

Although some people still think of meditation as being an exotic practice or something reserved for gurus, it is being recognized more and more for what it is: a natural, safe, accessible way to relieve tension and stress and to promote the healing of low back injuries and many other health conditions.

There are many ways to meditate, but regardless of the way you choose, the result, says Bernie Siegel, M.D., an expert on meditation, "is ultimately the same: to induce a restful trance which strengthens the mind by freeing it from its accustomed turmoil." In the process, meditation reduces or normalizes stress-hormone levels and evokes the relaxation response, a state of being in which heart rate, breathing rate, and blood pressure are reduced and tension is released, resulting in a reduction or elimination of aches and pains.

In a recent survey of more than 31,000 people conducted by the Centers for Disease Control and Prevention's National Center for Health Statistics, the researchers found that 62 percent of Americans had used some type of complementary or alternative therapy during the previous twelve months, and relief from back pain was one of the main reasons people sought such care. Nearly 8 percent of those surveyed said they had used meditation. A growing number of doctors and other health professionals, and even some health maintenance organizations (HMOs), have recognized the scientifically proven benefits of meditation in the treatment of pain, anxiety, depression, and high blood pressure, among other ailments.

One of the most popular and effective meditation techniques is mindfulness meditation, which was made popular in the United States by Jon Kabat-Zinn, Ph.D., who directs the Stress Reduction Program at the University of Massachusetts Medical School. It is certainly an approach that caught my attention and that of Natalia Morone, M.D., M.Sc., of the University of Pittsburgh Medical Center, a mindfulness meditation expert who offers programs in and does research with this form of meditation. A discussion of mindfulness meditation follows. Two other simple forms of meditation, breath meditation and walking meditation, are also discussed briefly.

Mindfulness Meditation

Mindfulness meditation involves focusing your attention on the present moment, allowing other thoughts, feelings, and sensations to pass by without thinking about them or judging them. It has been the subject of much research and has been found to be an excellent approach to dealing with chronic pain. Dr. Morone explains that mindfulness meditation helps you to become more aware of what is happening in your body and mind as it is occurring and gives you a new perspective on your pain.

"When you meditate, you're not thinking, 'I'm meditating to relieve the pain,'" says Dr. Morone. "That's not the point at all. You're meditating to be fully present in this moment and to be fully aware of what's going on in your body and your surroundings. With meditation you're training the mind to be present in the moment, and you begin to become aware of things, such as habits you may be doing that are harmful and may worsen your back pain."

Dr. Morone admits it sounds simple but emphasizes that the impact of meditation can be "profound," as she's witnessed in her practice and research. The different mindfulness techniques are the body scan and sitting and walking meditation. She explains how Stanley, a seventy-two-year-old retired landscape architect, was practicing the body scan meditation and made a startling discovery. He realized that a position he had been sitting in for decades while he read the newspaper every morning at his kitchen table was making his pain worse. It seemed like such a simple adjustment to make—he now doesn't slouch when he reads the newspaper—yet it made a world of difference.

"He had been completely unaware of it until he did the meditation and became conscious of what was going on in his body at that moment," says Dr. Morone. "That's what I mean about a new perspective and increased awareness of your pain."

Body Scan Technique

The body scan technique that I, Dr. Morone, and others have found to be so effective for helping people cope with chronic pain has been used very successfully for many years in the Stress Reduction Program at the University of Massachusetts Medical School and similar centers around the country. Regular practice of the body scan technique may result in a significant reduction in chronic pain.

In *Full Catastrophe Living* by Dr. Kabat-Zinn, he notes that practice of the body scan is where "our patients first learn to keep their attention focused over an extended period of time. It is the first technique they use to develop concentration, calmness, and mindfulness. . . . It is an excellent place for anyone to begin formal mindfulness meditation practice."

I can't leave this discussion of mindfulness and body scanning without telling one more story. Lloyd is an eighty-two-year-old World War II veteran who participated in Dr. Morone's mindfulness meditation program. When Lloyd first saw Dr. Morone, he could not stand for more than a minute without experiencing severe low back pain. When he walked, he used a cane. Lloyd was very excited because he had been invited to Europe to attend a special gathering of World War II veterans, but he was afraid he would not be able to cope with all the walking and standing such a trip and event involved. He started the meditation program one month before he was to leave on his trip and practiced the body scan regularly. He and Dr. Morone also discussed how he could use mindfulness meditation to help him cope with situations in which he might have to stand for an extended period of time.

Lloyd went to Europe with his cane. He forgot his cane on the airplane, had a marvelous time, and has not needed a cane since. What Lloyd had discovered while doing the body scan was that he was doing things that were making his back pain worse, such as carrying heavy groceries. Once he changed his habits, he found that his pain almost disappeared. Dr. Morone was extremely pleased with Lloyd's progress, and said, "I believe that his pain relief wasn't a direct effect of meditating on the pain but of meditating and understanding his behaviors."

The best way to learn and appreciate the power of the body scan is to participate in a mindfulness meditation program, but audiotapes are also available from various sources that can guide you at home (see the suggested reading and videos/DVDs section).

Breath Meditation

Breath meditation is one of the easiest and most effective ways to reduce tension in the body and, as recent (August 2005) research shows, to effectively manage chronic low back pain. In a study conducted at the Osher Center for Integrative Medicine, University of California, San Francisco, researchers evaluated the effectiveness of six to eight weeks (twelve sessions) of breath therapy versus physical therapy in thirty-six patients who had chronic low back pain. Testing during and after the study found that patients who participated in breathing therapy sessions improved significantly in terms of pain, function, and overall health, and that the changes were comparable with what those patients can expect from high-quality, long-term physical therapy. Thus, breathing therapy may be counted among the effective, noninvasive, nonpharmacological options for the management of chronic low back pain.

Breath meditation is easy to learn but requires practice, preferably daily, to get the most benefit. To begin, set aside about twenty minutes at a time and in a place where you won't be disturbed. Get comfortable; find a supportive chair or cushion that allows you to keep your spine relatively straight. If sitting is too painful, you may lie down, although falling asleep may be a problem. Be comfortable in your clothing as well: remove your shoes, loosen any tight clothing, and take off any jewelry that is distracting. Now you're ready to begin.

Focus your attention on your breathing. You may want to close your eyes, but notice how your breath moves into and out of your nose, your chest, and your abdomen. Don't try to change how you are breathing or force your breath; let it flow naturally. Some people find that breathing in through the nose and out through the mouth works best for them; others breathe only through the nose.

Keep your focus on your breath. If other thoughts creep into your mind, gently bring your focus back to your breathing. It is common for the mind to wander, so don't get anxious about it. Even very experienced meditators find that their mind sometimes wanders away from their focus.

Once you are comfortable focusing on your breath in your nose, chest, and/or abdomen, shift your attention to noticing how your breath feels in other parts of your body. Begin by focusing on the area just below your navel. As you take in a breath and let it out, notice how that area feels. You may or may not feel motion, tension, or tightness; either way, just be aware of the spot.

Now move your focus to your abdomen and concentrate on how your breath feels there. Remain focused on that site for a minute or two, then move on to your chest, your throat, and to the middle of your forehead, making sure to spend several minutes at each spot. (If you have more time to meditate, you can also focus on your toes, thighs, hands, arms, and/or shoulders.)

Once you have finished focusing on specific spots, turn your concentration to how your breath feels coming into and out of every pore in your entire body. Let your focus stay with this awareness for a minute or two, or as long as is comfortable. When you are ready, allow your attention to shift back to your surroundings. Take a deep breath, let it out slowly, and return to your day.

Walking Meditation

Despite its name, walking meditation is not designed as physical exercise. Rather, it combines relaxed movement with mindfulness, with emphasis on the meditation. This technique seems to work well for people who find sitting meditation to be too confining or who are more comfortable walking than sitting.

Walking meditation is usually done in a small space, a place where you can walk about twenty steps in either direction, unhindered by obstacles. This can be your office, a room in your house, your backyard, or your patio. Begin by closing your eyes; notice your breathing and how your body feels as you inhale and exhale. Focus on how your feet feel on the ground. Then open your eyes halfway; just enough so you can walk safely. Begin to walk slowly, paying attention to the sensations in your legs and how your feet move on the ground or floor. Your goal is to focus completely on the walking experience and on maintaining a straight spine.

When you reach your turnaround point, turn slowly and return to where you began, always being mindful of keeping your spine straight, how your feet feel on the ground, how your legs feel as you lift them, and how your weight shifts. If your mind strays from concentrating on your walking, gently bring it back, refocusing on the sensations associated with walking. Continue for about twenty minutes.

VISUALIZATION AND GUIDED IMAGERY

Do you like to daydream? Do you find yourself getting lost in your daydreams, losing track of time? Then visualization and guided imagery may be the tools for you. Visualization is a general term used to describe the use of various visual techniques to reduce pain, release stress and tension, and cope with different medical conditions. During visualization, people enter a state of relaxation and focus their attention on an image or images in their mind's eye. Guided imagery takes this exercise one step further: you move beyond one or two images and take a mental trip that incorporates many images and scenes, creating a story or a sequence of events that helps you achieve a specific goal; in this case, reducing back pain. For simplicity's sake, I will use the term *visualization* to refer to both methods.

Visualize This

You can learn visualization on your own from books or tapes, or you can work with a practitioner (e.g., psychiatrist, psychologist, master's-level counselor, nurse practitioner, or licensed social worker) who can help you through a few sessions until you feel ready to do it on your own. If you do work with a practitioner, it would be helpful to make a tape of the session(s) so you can review them at home.

Visualization is a personal experience: each person chooses images, situations, or scenes that are special for him or her. If you work with a practitioner, your sessions may be thirty to sixty minutes or even longer as you learn the process. At home, your sessions can be as short or long as you find useful, although many patients say that ten to twenty minutes is their average.

Here are some general preparation instructions, several brief visualizations, and one longer one. See the suggested reading and videos/DVDs section for other sources of information on visualization.

Preparation is simple: First, find a quiet spot where you won't be disturbed for your chosen amount of time. Get into a comfortable, relaxed position, and close your eyes if you want to. Then, concentrate on your breathing. You can use one of the breathing techniques discussed in the Breathing Therapy section. Continue with controlled breathing for several minutes until you feel relaxed; then begin your visualization exercise. You might choose one of the following brief visualizations, the longer guided imagery that follows, or something of your own:

- Imagine that you are getting an injection of morphine into the area that is painful for you. Visualize the drug spreading into the surrounding tissues, gradually eliminating your pain as it moves.
- Imagine that your pain is contained in a huge balloon, ready to burst. Now imagine that you have put a tiny

pinhole in the balloon, and the air is very slowly leaking out of the balloon. The air is your pain, and you hear it hissing out of the balloon, causing the balloon itself to ever so slowly collapse, relaxed, free of stress, tension, and pain.

- Imagine that your pain is a bright red light. It is shining all around you; perhaps it is making it impossible for you to see anything else. Now imagine that there is a dimmer light switch next to your hand. Place your hand on the switch and turn it slowly. As you do, the red light becomes less bright, and as the light begins to fade, your pain fades with it. Keep turning the switch until the light has completely gone out and you have extinguished all your pain with it.

- Imagine that you have put your back pain into a box. You are sitting in a chair, and the box is next to you; your pain is separate, not a part of you. Now imagine that the box is on a conveyer belt and is moving slowly away from you. You don't move; you sit in the chair, but the box moves away from you. It looks smaller and smaller to you until it disappears completely from sight.

Guided Imagery Exercise

The following guided imagery exercise can take about fifteen minutes to complete. Feel free to tape it or to use it as a model for something you create yourself, using different scenes and images. (I have used a forest scene as an example.) If you tape this exercise or develop one of your own, pause for five to ten seconds whenever you change a scene or introduce a new image. In the following exercise, I have used parentheses ( ) to indicate where you should pause when taping and during the exercise.

Begin with several minutes of controlled breathing until you feel relaxed. As you inhale, your mind becomes clearer and clearer ( ). Every time you exhale, your mind becomes lighter. Every breath you exhale contains molecules of tension that you are releasing into the atmosphere. Inhale and exhale slowly and gently, continuing to release tension with every exhale ( ).

Take a deep breath, and as you exhale, visualize a peaceful light in your mind ( ). Focus on the light and feel its warmth on your skin ( ). In your mind's eye you are walking toward the light ( ). With every inhale, you get closer to the light ( ); with every exhale, you release tension to the light. Continue to breathe gently and easily as you approach the light.

Continue walking toward the light until you pass through it, becoming one with the light ( ). As you imagine yourself in the midst of the light, stop and take a deep breath and welcome the warmth of the light ( ). Acknowledge that you are one with the light ( ).

Continue to breathe naturally and gently as you prepare to go on a journey ( ). You are walking in a meadow that is rich with wildflowers. Feel the flowers brush against your legs as you walk slowly ( ). Turn your face to the sun, and allow its warmth to wash over you ( ). As you inhale, enjoy the fragrance of the flowers ( ). As you exhale, send your tension and pain into the sky to rise above this bed of flowers.

Continue to breathe gently as you approach the forest ( ). Notice the butterflies flitting from flower to flower all around you ( ). Feel the moist earth under your feet ( ). Take a deep breath and acknowledge the fragrances once again ( ).

Ahead of you is a forest, thick with oak and maple and pine. Continue to walk toward it, and when you reach the spot where the meadow meets the trees, take a deep breath and welcome the coolness as you step into the shadows ( ). Listen for the birds singing overhead ( ). Notice how the leaves rustle in the branches as a breeze moves through the forest ( ). Feel the coolness of the breeze as it brushes over your skin ( ).

Continue to breathe gently and slowly as you walk deeper into the forest. Hear the fallen leaves crunch beneath your feet ( ); inhale the earthy aroma of the forest floor ( ); exhale your worries and tension ( ).

See how the sun breaks through the trees and creates dappled patterns on the forest floor ( ); feel the change in temperature on your skin as you pass through sun, then shadows ( ). Continue to breathe gently as you walk through the trees, reaching out to touch the bark of the oak ( ). Feel the roughness under your fingers. Place your palm on the trunk and imagine you can feel the pulsing of the life of the tree under your hand ( ).

Notice that the sun is breaking through the trees up ahead. Continue to walk slowly toward the light, listening to the birds overhead ( ). Take a deep breath as you step into the sunlight and out of the forest. Exhale your tension and pain as the sun warms you ( ). Take a deep breath and extend your arms over your head; slowly exhale as you bring your arms down slowly to your sides. Take a few more deep breaths as you prepare to reenter your world, relaxed ( ).

Practice this guided imagery or another one of your choice several times a day, and you should begin to experience less pain within a week or so, depending on your level of pain and whether you practice regularly. Some people find that there are one or two vivid scenes that work especially well at relieving their pain, and they can visualize them without having to go through the entire guided imagery exercise. Again, it will take some practice to reach this point, but once you do, you will have an effective tool to use against your pain.

What the Experts Say

Experts say that when it comes to imagining something and actually experiencing it, the brain reacts in the same way. Think about someone running his or her nails down a blackboard. Did you just feel a chill run through your spine? I did. That's because the brain's visual cortex, which processes images, works hand-in-hand with the autonomic nervous system, which controls involuntary functions, such as breathing and your responses to stress. The response of the visual cortex has been captured on positron emission tomography (PET), an imaging technique that can record brain activity. Studies show that the cerebral cortex is equally activated whether you actually experience something or you image it vividly.

Thus, when you expose yourself to pleasant images or situations, whether they are real or in your mind's eye, your body responds in positive ways—your pulse slows, your blood pressure declines, and your muscles relax. We know that stroking a dog or cat, for example, can reduce blood pressure, and it can have this effect whether you actually stroke the animal or you imagine doing so. Your body also releases such hormones as endorphins, which are natural painkillers.

When it comes to the impact of visualization on chronic pain, numerous researchers have looked for answers. A Purdue University School of Nursing study, for example, found that older women with chronic pain associated with osteoarthritis had a significant reduction in pain and mobility problems after participating in twice-daily guided imagery exercises when compared with women in a control group. A Kent State University study also found that guided imagery was effective in providing relief for patients with chronic pain. At the Cleveland Clinic Foundation, investigators found that guided imagery was effective in relieving chronic pain associated with tension headache.

Overall, visualization can be an effective way to cope with and manage chronic back pain. The more vivid the scenes or images you bring to mind, the more effective your visualization sessions will be.

IN CONCLUSION . . .

The power of the mind is an asset every individual has at his or her disposal to help change perspective, better understand the body, and manage pain. I believe that the psychologically based mind-body therapies discussed in this chapter can be as effective as medication if you are willing to take the time to learn and practice them. A little investment now in terms of time and energy can truly allow you to reap big benefits in a short time, and without the expense and side effects associated with drugs. Further information about all the therapies discussed in this chapter can be found using the resources and suggested reading sections.

Chapter 6

Step 4: Getting the Point: Injection Therapies

When the subject of injection therapy comes up during conversations with my patients, I sometimes see their apprehension as they mentally anticipate how it might feel to get an injection in their spine. I quickly reassure them, explaining that they will receive a local anesthetic to numb the site and perhaps a mild sedative to take the edge off any anxiety if necessary, and so the treatment can proceed relatively pain-free. If successful, which it often is, the injection treatment may provide them with months of low back pain relief, as well as a reprieve from leg, buttocks, or other referred pain they may have felt.

Those are months during which, ideally, they should take part in a physical therapy program recommended by their physician or physical therapist, one that includes a home exercise plan along with other treatments, such as any of those we've discussed in previous chapters. The addition of integrative, complementary treatments—massage, chiropractic, acupuncture, and visualization, for example—is important, because although injection therapies can provide relief from chronic low back pain, they are not a cure, and the relief may not be permanent. Rather, injection therapies are effective tools that are helpful primarily to facilitate rehabilitation and exercise therapy or, for some patients, as an alternative to systemic medications if they cannot tolerate or do not respond to such drugs. For patients who have a herniated disc that is accompanied by radiating pain, injection therapies often should be considered before other integrative therapies are tried.

In this chapter, I talk about some of the different types of localized injections my colleagues and I sometimes recommend to patients who have chronic back pain. In each case, I discuss the types of back pain these injections may help, how the treatment is delivered, what results can be expected, who is a good candidate for the treatment, and any associated side effects and complications.

AN INTRODUCTION TO INJECTION THERAPY

Spinal injections have been used to treat back pain since the early 1900s. Since then, new techniques and types of injections have been developed, and refinements are always in the works. Spinal injections actually have two important roles: back pain relief and as a diagnostic tool. For pain relief, because injection therapies can be delivered directly to the area that is generating the pain, they may be able to help patients avoid taking systemic painkillers that are often associated with many side effects. Depending on the type of injection and the cause of the pain, some injections can provide low back pain relief for a year or longer.

Injections are also used to help physicians identify which structure in the back is generating pain. For example, if your physician gives you an injection of lidocaine or a similar numbing medication and you experience temporary relief in the treated area (e.g., a sacroiliac joint or facet joint), this is a strong indication that a source (not necessarily the only source, however) of your pain has been found. Your physician can then take that information and consider it along with your history, the results of your physical examination, any test results, and your response to current or previous therapies to help him or her make a more accurate diagnosis and design a treatment plan for you.

If you and your physician discuss spinal injection therapy, make sure you get a clear understanding of what to expect, such as why he or she is suggesting the treatment(s) (e.g., pain relief, diagnostic, or both), what you can hope to gain, what preparations you will need to make before the procedure and arrangements for transportation after, and typical success rate.

EPIDURAL STEROID (CORTICOSTEROID) INJECTIONS

The most common type of localized injection for back pain is a lumbar epidural steroid (corticosteroid) injection. The injection can be done as an outpatient procedure, and side effects are minimal to none. Briefly, it involves injecting a potent anti-inflammatory substance into the epidural space that surrounds the spinal cord and spinal nerves in an effort to reduce any nerve swelling and thus relieve the accompanying pain. The goal of an epidural is to give patients fast relief from pain and inflammation so they can more actively participate in an exercise or rehabilitation program.

The Procedure

At the time you schedule your procedure, tell your doctor if you are taking any blood-thinning medications. He or she will tell you to stop them at an appropriate time and will also check your prothrombin time (a test of blood-clotting integrity) to make sure it is safe for you to undergo epidural injections. Also inform your physician if you develop any flulike symptoms before your appointment.

To prepare you for the epidural injection, the doctor—usually an anesthesiologist, pain specialist, physiatrist, or other physician who has been specially trained in the procedure—will inject a local anesthetic into the appropriate site, which may cause temporary burning and discomfort. Once the area is numb, the anesthesiologist will insert a needle into the epidural space and inject the steroid. This can be approached in one of two ways. The physician can feel your spine to guide him or her to the space where the needle should be injected; or, the preferred approach, X-ray fluoroscopy can be used to guide the needle directly into the epidural space or the neural foramen (the point where the root of the affected nerve leaves the spinal canal).

In either case, you will probably feel some pressure but no pain while the steroid is being administered. After the steroid has been injected, a small bandage will be placed on the injection site, and a nurse will check your blood pressure and pulse. Once the procedure is done, you will be allowed to rest for about thirty minutes, during which time a nurse will again monitor your blood pressure and pulse until they return to normal.

After the Procedure

You may return to your normal activities after the procedure, including any stretching or strengthening exercises, unless your doctor or physical therapist advises against it. It typically takes six to ten days to respond to the steroid. If you experience some soreness at the injection site, you can apply an ice pack to the area. If, however, the injection site becomes very tender, swollen, or red, contact your doctor.

Other side effects and complications are rare. Some patients experience temporary symptoms such as a rise in blood pressure; elevated blood glucose; fluid retention; or pain, numbness, or tingling that radiates from the origin of the pain. Very rare complications include meningitis, epidural abscess, hematoma, and adhesive arachnoiditis (an incurable inflammatory condition of the middle membrane of the spinal cord). A spinal headache can occur if the needle inadvertently penetrates the dural sac and causes cerebrospinal fluid to leak into the epidural area. Another rare occurrence is nerve root damage, although there is no risk of paralysis associated with this procedure.

Is an Epidural for You?

This procedure may be helpful if you have lower back pain that radiates into the leg and is caused by a herniated disc, spinal stenosis, degenerative disc disease, or other condition that causes compression, inflammation, and/or injury to a nerve root in the spine, such as diabetes, nerve root injury, or scarring from previous spinal surgery. Many patients, especially those who continue to do their back exercises and maintain good posture, are pain-free after just one injection. This result can last for weeks, months, and in some cases years. If you don't experience pain relief within two weeks of your first epidural injection, your doctor may suggest a second treatment. If you don't get results from a second injection, you are not likely to benefit from an epidural.

You are not a candidate for an epidural steroid injection if your pain is associated with a tumor or an infection. If either of these conditions is suspected, your physician should order an MRI scan to rule them out before proceeding with the injections.

FACET JOINT INJECTIONS

Facet joints are found along the entire length of your spine (see figure 1.1) and can become painful and stiff for various reasons, including trauma, inflammatory arthritis, and osteoarthritis. Twisting injuries, for example, can damage one or both facet joints, and the deterioration of cartilage associated with aging can also cause facet joint pain.

When the lumbar facet joints are involved, they can cause pain in the lower back, abdomen, legs, groin, or buttocks. People who have facet joint syndrome typically find it difficult to stand up straight or to get out of a chair, and they often walk hunched over, which compromises their center of gravity and places them at risk of falling.

If your doctor has completed a comprehensive physical examination and perhaps also ordered X-rays and suspects you have facet joint syndrome, he or she may suggest facet joint injections. Similar to epidural steroid injections, facet joint injections can be used to relieve pain and inflammation so you can tolerate and optimally benefit from physical therapy and exercise, but they are actually more helpful as a diagnostic aid—to identify the source of pain within the facet joints. Basically, if the injection relieves the pain, your doctor knows he or she has found a source (there could be more than one) of your pain.

The Procedure

Before the procedure, tell your doctor if you are taking blood thinners (including aspirin), if you are allergic to any anesthetics or iodine, or if you have heart problems. If you have high blood pressure, know that facet joint injections may raise it more. If you have diabetes, your blood sugar levels may rise. If you are taking medication for either of these conditions, you should continue your normal schedule. However, do not take any pain medications on the day of the procedure.

The procedure takes ten to thirty minutes. You will lie on your stomach on an X-ray table, and the injection site will be cleaned and numbed with medication, which will cause a stinging sensation for several seconds. Within a few minutes the site will be numb, at which time the doctor will direct a very small needle into the joints, using fluoroscopy (X-ray) to help guide the injection. First, a small amount of dye will be injected to make sure the needle is in the right place. Then, an anesthetic and a steroid will be injected. One or more joints may be treated, depending on the nature of your pain. You may feel some mild discomfort and pressure during the injection.

After the Procedure

Once the procedure is done, you will be asked to do something that is normally painful so you and your doctor can gauge how successful the injections have been. In most patients, some pain relief begins within fifteen minutes and continues to improve over the next few days, although it can take up to a week for significant relief to occur. You'll be given an evaluation sheet on which you will be asked to record the percentage of pain relief you experience during the week after the injection. Long-term (six months) pain relief is possible in 30 to 50 percent of patients who receive steroids in their facet joints. Infrequently, weakness or numbness in the legs occurs for a few hours after the injection, and the injection site may feel mildly irritated or numb for up to six or eight hours.

Is a Facet Joint Injection for You?

Evidence in the literature indicates that facet joint injections have more value as a diagnostic tool than as an effective pain reliever. One recent study notes that the success rate for these injections ranges from 18 to 63 percent, although some studies show they provide no significant relief. Thus, the use of lumbar facet joint injections for the treatment of chronic low back pain remains controversial.

Another factor to consider is that for some patients, facet joint syndrome is chronic, and so they get only short-term relief from injections. For these patients, a procedure called radiofrequency rhizotomy is an option. Radiofrequency rhizotomy involves focusing radio waves on the nerves that arise from the facet joints. These nerves transmit pain signals to the brain, and heating them with radio waves blocks these signals. The pain relief may last from six months to two years.

TRIGGER-POINT INJECTIONS

I talked about trigger points earlier, during our discussion of myofascial pain, so it's no surprise that trigger-point injections are indicated in treating low back pain associated with myo-fascial pain syndrome. Like the other injection therapies discussed in this chapter, trigger-point injections are most effective in allowing you to pursue your physical therapy or rehabilitation. Unlike other injection therapies discussed here, however, trigger-point injections are delivered to muscle rather than to a nerve root or joint.

The Procedure

Trigger-point injections can be done in your doctor's office. The injections themselves usually take only five to ten minutes. Before you receive the injections, the chosen area will be numbed. Some physicians use a massage method called spray and stretch (see chapter 7) to help relax and stretch the muscle(s) to be treated. The injections can be administered in several ways. Although some physicians choose to inject steroids, I believe it is best to inject a local anesthetic alone, as steroids can cause muscle wasting, dimpling, and loss of pigmentation in the skin. In fact, trigger-point injections and "dry needling" (insertion of a needle such as an acupuncture needle into a trigger point without injecting any substance) are both effective therapies, as both cause the local twitch response—a rapid contraction and relaxation of the muscle when the needle is inserted. Unfortunately, however, the vast majority of third-party providers will reimburse for trigger-point treatments only when a steroid and/or anesthetic is injected.

After the Procedure

Once the injections are done and the monitoring devices have been removed, you will be free to leave. You will only need to have someone drive you home if you elected to take a sedative. You can resume your normal activities unless your doctor tells you otherwise, and avoid excessive use of the treated muscle for a day or two. Side effects are usually minor and may include temporary localized pain and bruising. Rare complications include infection and inadvertent, temporary numbing of the spine.

Are Trigger-Point Injections for You?

Reports on the effectiveness of trigger-point injections vary: some studies show significant results, while others are not clear, or their findings are mixed. Thus, a decision to try these injections must be made on a case-by-case basis. For some patients, injections may be more appropriate when they are given before physical therapy sessions start; other patients may begin rehabilitation, and then their physical therapist will recommend trigger-point injections because he or she believes the pain is jeopardizing compliance and/or progress with physical therapy. Patients who are not good candidates for systemic medications also may benefit from trigger-point injections. If you and your doctor decide you should try trigger-point injections, they should be viewed as a complement to your regular exercise program. Your doctor should also monitor your exercise progress and any pain or discomfort that you experience in the months after the injections.

SACROILIAC JOINT INJECTION

The sacroiliac joint is next to the spine and connects the bottom of the spine (sacrum) with the pelvis. According to a 2004 study, pain in the sacroiliac joint is the cause of 15 percent of cases of chronic low back pain. Those cases include individuals who have experienced trauma, strained ligaments (from overuse), or hypermobility or who have osteoarthritis. Sacroiliac joint injections can be helpful both diagnostically and therapeutically, especially when used in combination with a physical therapy program. The sacroiliac joint is complicated and can become painful because of problems with the spine (e.g., scoliosis), legs (e.g., hip and/or knee arthritis, leg length discrepancy), or pelvis (e.g., problems with the pelvic muscles). Thus, injecting the sacroiliac joint without addressing the underlying problem that caused the painful joint will nearly always result in only temporary pain reduction.

In fact, pain in the hip and/or knee joints is not uncommon among people who have chronic low back pain associated with the sacroiliac joint. When one or both of these key areas are painful, people often modify their gait to compensate, and eventually, sacroiliac joint pain can result. Therefore, these individuals can benefit from receiving injection therapy in the hip and/or knee to ward off or treat sacroiliac joint pain.

Identifying sacroiliac joint pain can be challenging because it radiates to different sites in the body, especially the thigh, but also to the foot, groin, and abdomen. Thus, it's necessary to differentiate it from other common causes of chronic low back pain, including facet joint pain, myofascial pain, and degenerative disc disease. I can get several good indications of sacroiliac joint involvement by, say, noting any pain when I place stress on the joint or by taking leg length measurements to see if there is a discrepancy, as such a difference can cause sacroiliac joint pain.

Preparation for sacroiliac joint injections is similar to that for epidural and facet joint injections. The physician uses a fluoroscope to guide the needle and then inserts it into the sacroiliac joint to inject lidocaine and a steroid. Sacroiliac joint injections may be repeated about every sixteen weeks. Post-injection care is similar to that of epidural and facet joint injections, with physical therapy and a regular exercise program beginning (or continuing from preprocedure) within a day or two.

Giving the injection itself is often diagnostic. Physicians generally agree that pain in the sacroiliac joint is the cause of a person's lower back pain if the injection results in a reduction in pain greater than 75 percent. If the injection results in less than a 50 percent reduction in pain, the sacroiliac joint probably is not the source of the pain.

Stephen's Story

When Stephen first came to my office in February of 2005, he had been suffering with lower back pain and leg pain for fifteen years. The pain began when he was fifty and was working as an architect for a large design firm. The pain started as a dull ache in his lower back, and it progressively grew sharper and soon radiated down his right leg and was accompanied by tingling and occasional numbness in the leg. Standing and walking made the pain worse, sometimes a 7 or 8 out of 10. He went to see a physiatrist and received epidural injections, but they did not help. In 1996, he underwent laminec-tomy, which provided some relief, leaving him with a pain level of 2 or 3 out of 10.

Then in 2000, the pain increased in intensity and also affected his left leg. Again the pain was about a 7 or 8 out of 10 at its worst and 2 to 3 out of 10 at its best. He underwent another surgery in 2002, and for about one month the pain was minimal, but it returned "with a vengeance" after that time. He became depressed and his doctor prescribed clonazepam (Klonopin) for anxiety, bupropion (Wellbutrin) for depression, and zolpidem (Ambien) for sleep. He reported that the pain remained at 3 out of 10 at its least and 8 out of 10 at its worst over the next two years. He was also experiencing some tingling and numbness in both legs, but it was worse in the right leg. Again, the symptoms were worse when standing and walking, and he got some relief when he sat down or pulled his knees up to his chest. To deal with the pain, his doctor prescribed the combination drug acetaminophen and oxycodone (Percocet) to take as needed. Stephen was about twenty-five pounds overweight at that time, so he met with a dietician to help him lose weight, which he hoped would relieve some of the pressure on his lower back. He lost thirty pounds, but he said it didn't seem to have any impact on his back pain.

When Stephen first came to see me, he said his pain was 6 out of 10 most of the time. During an intensive examination, I detected muscle spasm on both sides of the spine, greater on the right than on the left, as well as spasms of the left piriformis muscle. Stephen's sacroiliac joints were tender, and he experienced pain when he extended his back, but not when he flexed it. Based on these and other findings, and the fact that he had had several surgeries, I diagnosed Stephen with failed back surgery syndrome that was complicated by lumbar spinal stenosis, myofascial pain, sacroiliac joint syndrome, and scoliosis. I prescribed physical therapy, which included a comprehensive home exercise program, and short-term use of opioids, and his pain improved. However, he still had moderate pain in his right sacroiliac joint which both prevented him from benefiting fully from his exercise program and from sleeping adequately, so I referred him for sacroiliac joint injections, which were very successful. Stephen has stopped taking the opioids and only rarely needs his sleeping pills. As part of his "therapy," he has taken up line dancing at the local community center with his wife and is able to walk a mile several times a week with minimal or no discomfort.

PROLOTHERAPY

Prolotherapy, also sometimes referred to as sclerosant therapy or sclerotherapy, is used to treat degenerative disc disease, sacroiliac problems, and sciatica. The idea behind prolotherapy differs somewhat from other injection therapies. Advocates of prolotherapy believe that some back pain is caused by damaged or weakened ligaments and/or tendons. Ligaments and tendons generally have a poor blood supply, which means they have a more difficult time healing after injury. Incomplete healing causes the ligaments and tendons to weaken, and they become a source of chronic pain.

To strengthen and repair these structures, repeated injections with irritant solutions (typically a mixture of dextrose, glycerol, phenol, and lidocaine) are given to intentionally cause inflammation at the chosen site. The inflammation in turn stimulates natural healing, with the intended end result being stronger ligaments and/or tendons and reduced pain. A course of treatment typically involves four to six treatments at four- to six-week intervals, which allows time for the growth of new connective tissue. Healing usually takes about six weeks after the initial treatment.

Prolotherapy studies reportedly have so far produced good results. A recent Canadian retrospective case review evaluated 177 patients who had chronic spinal pain and who received prolotherapy injections (dextrose and lidocaine) weekly for up to three weeks. The patients were followed up for a period ranging from two months to two and a half years. Ninety-one percent of the patients said they had less pain, 85 percent said they were better able to take part in daily activities, and 84 percent said their ability to work had improved. No one reported any complications from the injections. The results sound promising, but they would be more convincing if they were derived from a controlled trial.

A more scientific study was done in Australia, where a randomized, partially blinded, controlled study evaluated 110 patients who were treated for six months and then followed for up to two years. The patients were assigned to receive either prolotherapy (glucose and lidocaine) or normal saline, and then were assigned to an exercise program or to normal activity. In terms of pain relief and reduced disability, prolotherapy injections were not significantly more effective than saline, and the type of activity did not seem to add to or detract from the results. Thus, the benefit seems to come from the injection itself and the response it stimulates in the body, and not the substance injected.

Two other studies reported that prolotherapy was superior to placebo injections. In one of those studies, published in 1993 in the *Journal of Spinal Disorders*, 77 percent of the patients reported an improvement of 50 percent or more in back pain, compared with only 52 percent of the patients who received a placebo.

INTRADISCAL ELECTROTHERMAL ANNULOPLASTY

Intradiscal electrothermal annuloplasty (IDEA), also referred to as intradiscal electrothermal therapy (IDET), is a procedure in which a wire is inserted into a disc and heat is applied, which destroys the nerves. The heat also causes the proteins in the disc walls to reshape and gradually strengthen. The procedure cannot be done if the disc is severely deteriorated. I decided to include IDEA in this chapter even though it is not an injection procedure because it involves the use of a fluoroscopically guided catheter to help administer the heat to the disc.

This is a relatively new procedure, but it is already showing some promise in the treatment of chronic low back pain, especially as an alternative to spinal fusion in patients who need one or two discs fused. In a study conducted by David A. Bryce, M.D., and his colleagues, for example, eighty-six patients with chronic low back pain underwent the procedure at a temperature of 90°C for an average of fifteen minutes and were then evaluated for pain and disability at various points post-treatment. At six months, fifty-one patients had significant improvement in pain and functioning, and at one year, the same was true for the thirty-three patients who remained in the study. The researchers noted, however, that although the women in the study continued to benefit from the procedure beyond the three- to six-month period, the men did not. The reason for this difference between men and women is not yet understood.

In another study, fifty-eight patients who had not improved after undergoing other aggressive nonsurgical treatments were treated with IDEA and then evaluated at least two years later. The patients reported a significant improvement in both pain and function, as well as an improvement in quality of life. In yet another study, thirty-three patients underwent IDEA and were reevaluated at a mean of fifteen months after treatment. Seventy percent of the patients reported complete (24 percent) or partial (46 percent) pain relief.

Yet not all is rosy with IDEA. Investigators at the Spine Institute at Saint John's Health Center, Santa Monica, California, followed up with thirty-eight patients who had undergone IDEA one year previously and asked about their postprocedure experiences. Half (50 percent) were dissatisfied with the results, fourteen (37 percent) were satisfied, and five (13 percent) were undecided. Fifteen (39 percent) had less pain after the procedure, eleven (29 percent) had more pain, and eleven (29 percent) had no change. When they were asked about their medication use after IDEA, eleven (29 percent) used more pain medication, ten (26 percent) used the same, twelve (32 percent) used less, and five (13 percent) stopped using medication.

IN CONCLUSION . . .

Injection therapies are typically used for two reasons: for relatively quick, temporary pain relief as a way to facilitate successful physical therapy and to help with diagnosis. When a patient has a herniated disc associated with pain radiating down the leg, epidural injections alone may be useful. Use of injection therapies may also eliminate or reduce a patient's need for oral medications, which are typically associated with undesirable side effects.

Chapter 7

―――――――― ❧ ――――――――

Step 5: Meet the Meds

If you are taking any kind of drugs for your back pain, I strongly recommend you familiarize yourself with what is known about them. After all, the use of pain medications is often the first and only option offered by many doctors to their patients who have chronic back pain. I, however, view the use of pain-relief medications as *one option, to be used judiciously, as a means to an end. That end is improved function so patients can optimize and comply with rehabilitation efforts. I also believe that if you do take pain-relief medications, you should also use non-pharmacological approaches as discussed in previous steps, with the goal of trying to phase out or at least reduce the intake of medications once the other options provide sufficient relief.*

These are not unattainable goals. In fact, they are a routine part of my philosophy and practice, and I am happy to say that more and more patients are able to realize these goals as they learn about the various complementary and integrative medicine options at their disposal, like those discussed in previous chapters. As you've seen, these are goals you can reach if you are willing to explore and embrace alternatives to medications. And while it's true that some of these alternatives are not covered by insurance providers, thus forcing patients to pay out-of-pocket (which many cannot afford to do), if they want to pursue them, it is also true that other alternatives such as exercise—typically the most effective alternative—and various mind-body techniques we discussed can be done with little to no expense.

At the same time, however, I am fully aware that medications are still very much a part of the popular treatment strategy for chronic low back pain. The fact is, most patients come to me with a history of medication use, and I cannot ask them to simply stop taking their drugs. And for good reasons: many drugs cause serious withdrawal symptoms if they are stopped abruptly, and I need to provide these individuals with safe, effective pain-relieving alternatives. Drugs do have their place; I am not saying they should be banned from everyone's treatment plan. But I do believe, and continue to witness in my practice, that *medication use can sometimes be dramatically reduced, modified to include drugs that are less toxic, or even entirely eliminated.*

Which drugs are doctors prescribing to treat chronic back pain? What should you know about them if your doctor recommends one or more for you? If you need medication to help you through the beginning stages of physical therapy and an exercise program, which ones should you consider? Which drugs provide the most benefit with the least risk? Which over-the-counter (OTC) drugs are effective pain relievers?

In this chapter, I talk about three categories of medications that are used to treat chronic back pain: topical and OTC systemic medications, nonopioid (non-narcotic) prescription medications (e.g., NSAIDs, antidepressants, anticonvulsants), and opioids (narcotics). We look at how they work; expected results; side effects; who should avoid them and when; typical dosages; available forms; how older patients may react to them; and how they may interact with other drugs, herbal remedies, and foods.

TOPICAL PREPARATIONS

Topical pain-relieving preparations are applied to the skin as gels, ointments, creams, or sprays and are available both OTC and by prescription. Although they are used primarily to treat acute pain, they can provide some temporary relief for chronic low back pain by helping reduce inflammation under the skin or by blocking the transmission of nerve signals, especially before and after exercise and physical therapy sessions.

Types of Topical Pain Medications

There are two common types of topical pain relievers: analgesics and local anesthetics. Topical analgesics include NSAID preparations that help reduce swelling and inflammation of soft tissues. Some of these include a formula that contains diclofenac (Voltaren) and others that contain trolamine salicylate, found in several OTC products (e.g., Aspercreme, Myoflex, and Sportscreme). Another type of topical preparation contains capsaicin, the chemical in chili peppers that makes them hot. When capsaicin cream is applied to the skin, it causes a burning sensation that some people find mildly unpleasant. It is believed that this burning depletes nerve cells of a chemical called substance P, which plays a role in transmitting pain signals. Some patients get relief using capsaicin cream (e.g., Dolorac, Zostrix), although it usually takes about two weeks of applying the cream three to four times a day before the benefit is apparent.

Topical local anesthetics such as benzocaine, lidocaine, and tetracaine can be effective against chronic pain. Specifically, I have prescribed a lidocaine patch for some patients who have localized myofascial pain, and they have generally been happy with the results. The problem with this patch is that it is expensive, and therefore many insurance companies will not pay for it.

One type of topical anesthetic can be helpful when you are preparing for sessions of physical therapy and exercise. This spray anesthetic and how it is used are discussed below (see Vapocoolant: Spray and Stretch).

Topical pain relievers should not be used without first consulting your physician. Never apply these medications to broken or inflamed skin or if you have eczema. Talk to your doctor before using a topical medication if you have severe liver or kidney disease, asthma, glucose-6-phosphate dehydrogenase deficiency, or an intolerance for certain oral medications. If a rash or other allergic reaction develops, stop using the drug and contact your doctor at once.

Vapocoolant: Spray and Stretch

One local anesthetic used especially for patients who have myofascial pain is a skin refrigerant, or vapocoolant, used during a therapeutic process called spray and stretch. In our previous discussion of myofascial pain (see chapter 1), I noted that it is possible to relieve muscle pain by stretching the muscle and restoring it to its normal length. However, the stretching itself may be painful, and it can be helpful in some cases to temporarily block the pain receptors while the muscle is being stretched. Some ways to accomplish this include myofascial massage (chapter 4), trigger-point injections (chapter 6), and spray and stretch. This latter technique is helpful for patients who cannot tolerate acupressure to their trigger points and/or do not want or cannot tolerate injections. On the other hand, many patients tolerate gentle stretching quite well, especially when performed by a skilled therapist. For these patients, it is not necessary to block the pain receptors prior to stretching.

If the therapist chooses to use spray and stretch, he or she may first apply a heating pad or moist heat to the affected area for about five minutes. The therapist then will spray the skin with the vapocoolant in a sweeping motion in the direction of the pain pattern. The therapist then will apply pressure to the trigger point, gently stretching the muscle, and then may spray on more vapocoolant or apply more heat. Depending on which muscle is being treated, the therapist may also include some range-of-motion exercises. This sequence of spray and stretch is repeated several times until the muscle is relaxed but not overstretched.

NONOPIOID MEDICATIONS

The category of nonopioid drugs, both prescription and OTC, includes a varied and sizeable group of medications that are often used to treat and manage chronic low back pain. Along with analgesics (pain relievers), this category of medications also consists of drugs traditionally used to treat other conditions, including depression, insomnia, and seizures, but which have been found to be useful in addressing chronic pain symptoms.

Acetaminophen

Acetaminophen (such as Tylenol) is an analgesic and antipyretic (fever reducing) medication that is the primary member of the drug group called *p*-aminophenol derivatives. It is as effective as aspirin when it comes to reducing pain and fever, but it has no anti-inflammatory abilities. Therefore, if inflammation is a contributing factor in your back pain, acetaminophen alone will not be sufficient. For this reason, many people use both acetaminophen and an NSAID (see Nonsteroidal Anti-Inflammatory Drugs in this chapter). This combination can be especially helpful during the early stages of an exercise and/or physical therapy program but should be taken only with your doctor's guidance.

The usual dose of acetaminophen is 325 to 1,000 mg every four to six hours, and you should never exceed 4,000 mg daily. You can expect to experience acetaminophen's painkilling benefits within thirty to sixty minutes of taking the drug, and you don't have to worry about developing tolerance (a loss of the drug's pain-relieving benefits), even with prolonged use. An advantage of acetaminophen is that, unlike many other pain-relieving drugs, its use is not associated with gastrointestinal problems. If, however, you have liver problems, you definitely should not exceed a total daily dose of 2,000 mg, and in fact in such cases, I recommend you avoid this drug altogether.

Some people become lax when using acetaminophen because it is readily available OTC and is inexpensive, a combination that lulls them into believing it is a harmless drug. Acetaminophen is cleared through the liver, and so the potential for harm to this organ exists if the drug is taken in excessive amounts (more than 4,000 mg daily for adults). Liver damage can also occur if you take acetaminophen along with the herbs chaparral, comfrey, or coltsfoot. Alcohol and acetaminophen are not a good mix, as alcohol increases the risk of liver toxicity and liver failure. The best advice is, if you're taking acetaminophen, don't drink alcohol. Taking high doses of vitamin C (3,000 mg or more daily) along with acetaminophen can raise the levels of the drug in the body and increase the risk of drug toxicity. Chronic use of acetaminophen can damage the kidneys.

Nonsteroidal Anti-Inflammatory Drugs

The drug class nonsteroidal anti-inflammatory drugs (NSAIDs) consists of many products, both OTC and prescription, for addressing the inflammation, stiffness, pain, and tenderness associated with back pain. The main benefit of NSAIDs is their ability to reduce the activity of cyclooxygenase (COX), enzymes that make prostaglandins, with the result being a decrease in prostaglandin production. This is desirable because prostaglandins promote inflammation and sensitize peripheral nerve endings, two situations involved in pain.

There are several subtypes of NSAIDs, which I list in the table on page 208. All of them work in similar ways to reduce COX activity, although the amount of time they are effective before another dose is required varies significantly (see the table), and this has an impact on compliance. The NSAIDs also share some other characteristics. One is the catch-22 factor: NSAIDs are more effective when they are taken regularly over time, yet long-term use exposes you to potential risks and complications. Among them is the risk of kidney damage. If you take an NSAID on a regular basis, your doctor will want to take a blood test periodically to monitor your kidney function.

As a precaution, NSAIDs should be taken with food to minimize any chance of stomach upset. The risk of gastrointestinal problems is always a concern, although less so if you are using a newer NSAID, a COX-2 inhibitor, which are discussed below. Other potential risks should be discussed with your doctor before you take any NSAID if you have the following conditions or situations: heart disease, thyroid problems, diabetes, intolerance to aspirin or other NSAIDs or pain relievers, high blood pressure, if you are pregnant or breast-feeding, or if you normally consume three or more alcoholic beverages daily. NSAIDs have a blood-thinning effect that is more dominant in some drugs than in others (e.g., ibuprofen has a greater tendency for thinning the blood than does naproxen). Therefore, taking an NSAID may reduce the effectiveness of any blood pressure medications you are using. Use of herbs that affect clotting, such as clove oil, feverfew, garlic, ginkgo, and ginseng, also should be avoided when taking an NSAID.

Potentially serious side effects may result if NSAIDs are used along with other drugs. For example, simultaneous use of aspirin increases the risk of serious side effects, while ibuprofen use may decrease the effects of hydralazine, captopril, beta-blockers, furosemide, and thiazides. NSAIDs may also increase the risk of toxicity of methotrexate and phenytoin. Generally, you should never take more than one brand of NSAID at a time.

Deciding which NSAID is best for your needs is largely a personal choice. Many patients make that choice based on cost, convenience, and effectiveness, and for those reasons, ibuprofen and naproxen are commonly used because they are available over-the-counter, are relatively inexpensive, and produce good results. The prescription COX-2 inhibitors were popular because of their reduced risk of gastrointestinal complications. However, two of the three on the market were withdrawn in 2004 and 2005, and the fate of the remaining product was uncertain as of late 2005 (see COX-2 Inhibitors below).

NSAID Subtypes

Drug (Generic, Brand Name[s])	Usual Dose (mg)	Dosing (hrs)
Aspirin	650	Every 4–6 hrs
Choline magnesium trisalicylate (Trilisate)	500–750	8–12
Diflunisal (Dolobid)	1,000, then 500	8–12
Etodolac (Lodine)	200–400	6–8
Flurbiprofen (Ansaid)	50–100	8–12
Ibuprofen (Advil, Motrin, Nuprin)	400–600	6–8
Indomethacin (Indocin)	25	8–12
Ketoprofen (Orudis)	25–50	6–8
Meclofenamate (Meclomen)	50–100	4–6
Nabumetone (Relafen)	500–1,000	12–24
Naproxen (Aleve, Naprosyn)	250–500	12
Naproxen (Anaprox)	550, then 275	12
Oxaprozin (Daypro)	1,200	24
Piroxicam (Feldene)	20	24
Salsalate (Disalcid)	500–1,000	8–12
Sulindac (Clinoril)	150–200	12
Tolmetin (Tolectin)	200–600	8

COX-2 inhibitors (e.g., celecoxib [Celebrex]) are among the newest additions to the NSAID family and, at the same time, the ones most subject to controversy. Some advantages of COX-2 inhibitors over other NSAIDs are that they are less likely to cause gastrointestinal complications and they do not hinder blood clotting, which makes them safer for patients who take blood thinners. However, of the three that were approved by the Food and Drug Administration (FDA) (celecoxib, rofecoxib [Vioxx], and valdecoxib [Bextra]), only the first one remained available on the market as of mid 2006. That's because studies showed their use potentially increases the risk for cardiovascular events such as heart attack and stroke, which caused the FDA to withdraw Vioxx and Bextra from the market (2004 and 2005, respectively). A National

Cancer Institute study, called the Adenoma Prevention with Celecoxib trial, was halted in December 2004 because an independent analysis found a 2.5-fold increased risk in fatal and nonfatal cardiovascular events among subjects in the study. This finding was not enough to have celecoxib withdrawn from the market, however. If you are currently using celecoxib or have thought about using it, you and your physician should discuss the risks and benefits. You can also visit the celecoxib Web site for the latest information (www.celebrex.com).

Muscle Relaxants

Unlike the other drugs I discuss in this chapter, muscle relaxants are not a separate class of drugs but rather a group of various medications from different classes—namely, benzodiazepines, nonbenzodiazepines, and antispasmodics. These drugs are believed to work by suppressing the activity of nerves in the brain and spinal cord (the central nervous system) and can cause serious reactions.

Typically, physicians prescribe muscle relaxants for short-term use to relieve low back pain associated with muscle spasms. Their effectiveness is questionable, however, especially for treatment of chronic pain, and they are associated with significant side effects (see examples below). Drowsiness, for example, affects up to 30 percent of people who take muscle relaxants. No studies have found muscle relaxants to provide better relief than NSAIDs. Thus, if you feel you need to take medication, you should discuss with your doctor the risks and benefits of taking a muscle relaxant as compared with another analgesic such as acetaminophen or an NSAID.

Muscle relaxants may also have negative results when taken along with some of the common herbal remedies on the market. In particular, herbs that produce sedative effects, such as calendula, catnip, goldenseal, gotu kola, hops, lady's slipper, passionflower, skullcap, St. John's wort, and valerian, among others, may increase the severity of the sedative reactions.

Several muscle relaxants are commonly prescribed for low back pain. Consult your physician about these and any other muscle relaxant he or she may prescribe.

- **Carisoprodol** (Rela, Soma). This drug may be habit-forming, especially if it is taken with any drugs that affect the mind, including alcohol. Side effects include extreme weakness, loss of balance, vision problems, agitation, irritability, headache, depression, insomnia, rapid heartbeat, flushing, vomiting, hiccups, increased tissue swelling, rash, dizziness, nausea, and allergic reactions. The usual dosage is 350 mg every eight hours, as needed. If you suddenly stop taking carisoprodol, you may experience headache and insomnia.

- **Cyclobenzaprine** (Flexeril). This drug is chemically related to some antidepressants, although it does not have antidepressant characteristics. The usual dosage is 10 mg every six hours, or it can be taken before going to bed to help with sleep problems. Side effects include dry mouth, drowsiness, euphoria, depression, headache, nightmares, dizziness, numbness, tingling, vision problems, and seizures.

- **Diazepam** (Valium). This benzodiazepine can be highly addictive. If your doctor prescribes diazepam, you should take it for no more than two weeks, as it can change your sleep cycles and make it very hard for you to sleep once you stop taking the drug. Long-term use of diazepam can cause depression. The most common side effect is drowsiness, but it also is associated with clumsiness, extreme weakness, breathing difficulties, slow heartbeat, disturbed vision, confusion, slurred speech, and tremor. The typical dosage is 5 to 10 mg every six hours, as needed to relieve pain.

- **Baclofen** (Lioresal). Baclofen is a commonly prescribed muscle relaxant. It is available in tablets and usually is given at a dose of 15 mg daily for the first few days of treatment, then increased by your doctor to 40 to 80 mg daily. Among older patients, it is more likely to cause mood changes, severe drowsiness, hallucinations, depression, and confusion than it is among younger individuals.

A 2005 review of thirty trials of the use of muscle relaxants in people who had low back pain found that overall, these drugs relieved pain symptoms of acute low back pain in the short term, but their benefits for relieving chronic pain were less convincing. The reviewers also reported that the incidence of side effects was consistently high for both benzodiazepines and nonbenzodiazepines, and that combining muscle relaxants with NSAIDs speeded up recovery but also increased the risk for dizziness, drowsiness, and other central nervous system side effects. This finding suggests that if you feel the need to take medication, you may want to opt for an alternative analgesic over a muscle relaxant, and especially avoid taking both a muscle relaxant and an NSAID.

Antidepressants

As I mentioned previously, the presence of chronic pain can cause depression, and when you are depressed, you are less able to cope with pain or to feel motivated to stay with an exercise program. Therefore, I believe it is important to treat depression and pain simultaneously to help ensure success with a pain-relief program. Basically, there are three classes of antidepressants to consider: tricyclic antidepressants (e.g., amitriptyline [Elavil], nortriptyline [Pamelor], imipramine [Tofranil]), which are the older of the three groups and work by preventing the uptake of the brain neurotransmitters norepinephrine and serotonin; selective serotonin reuptake inhibitors (SSRIs), which have an impact on serotonin and include sertraline (Zoloft), paroxetine (Paxil), fluoxetine (Prozac), escitalopram (Lexapro), and citalopram (Celexa); and serotonin-norepinephrine reuptake inhibitors (SNRIs), which inhibit the reuptake of both serotonin and norepinephrine and include duloxetine (Cymbalta) and venlafaxine (Effexor).

The tricyclic antidepressants are associated with many common side effects, including but not limited to dizziness, drowsiness, headache, nausea, tiredness, weakness, blurry vision, dry mouth, constipation, increased appetite, weight gain, and impaired urination. The use of tricyclic antidepressants can also make certain conditions worse, including asthma, bipolar disorder, blood disorders, convulsions, enlarged prostate, glaucoma, heart disease, high blood pressure, hyperthyroidism, stomach or intestinal problems, and kidney or liver disease.

If you are taking an antihypertensive medication, adding a tricyclic antidepressant may cause low blood pressure. Similarly, if you are taking any central nervous system depressants, such as other types of antidepressants, tranquilizers, or sleeping aids, the effects of the tricyclic medications may increase. Tricyclic antidepressants also should not be combined with herbal supplements such as hops, kava, passionflower, St.

John's wort, valerian, SAMe, and 5-HTP. You also should avoid taking the tricyclics with grapefruit or grapefruit juice.

Generally, I am cautious if I prescribe tricyclics to my older patients, as side effects such as drowsiness, dizziness, confusion, dry mouth, vision problems, constipation, and urination difficulties may impose a greater risk in older patients than in younger ones. These reactions are less common with lower doses of the drugs.

Side effects associated with SSRIs and SNRIs include anxiety, nausea, diarrhea, headache, insomnia, weight gain, sweating, impotence, and loss of libido. These reactions tend to be less intense with SNRIs. If SSRIs or SNRIs are taken along with other medications that inhibit the reuptake of serotonin, patients may develop serotonin syndrome, which is a medical emergency. Symptoms associated with serotonin syndrome include (but are not limited to) euphoria, drowsiness, restlessness, clumsiness, sweating, muscle twitching, fever, confusion, shivering, and diarrhea. Loss of consciousness and death may occur.

OPIOIDS

Opioids are very potent pain relievers that are derived from or resemble those derived from the opium plant and include codeine, morphine, oxycodone, fentanyl, and meperidine, among others. Until recently, opioids were used almost exclusively to treat acute severe pain and pain associated with cancer. Nonmalignant chronic pain, such as chronic low back pain, was thought to be unresponsive to these drugs, or their use was thought to be too risky.

Much of that thinking has changed among medical professionals. Several recent studies by pain specialists, for example, support the safety and effectiveness of the use of opioids by patients who have chronic nonmalignant pain, although the controversy continues because of their potential for addiction and the risk of significant side effects.

A Look at the Risks

Before I discuss the risks associated with the use of opioids, I think it's important for you to understand what I mean when I talk about *dependence*, *addiction*, and *tolerance*, as these terms are often misunderstood and even used incorrectly by the media and some health professionals. According to the National Library of Medicine, *drug dependence (addiction)* is the compulsive use of a substance even though such use results in negative consequences that can be severe or even life-threatening. Dependence can cause long-lasting chemical changes in the brain and result in physical and/or psychological damage. Physical dependence means you need a drug to function, while psychological dependence is an overwhelming desire to continue using the drug either because of the pleasurable experience it provides, because it helps you better cope with negative life experiences, or other psychological reasons. Physiological dependence is a reversible state that develops in the body after a person has been taking an opioid for a period of time and is the reason that opioids need to be tapered (i.e., the dose gradually reduced) rather than stopped abruptly. By gradually reducing the opioid dose, symptoms of withdrawal can be avoided. *Tolerance* is a state in which you need greater and greater doses of the drug to obtain the same pain-relief benefits you got initially.

For people who have significant chronic pain, I don't believe addiction is a problem when taking opioids. In fact, the risk of true addiction is believed to be less than one in two hundred. If your physician monitors your progress carefully and proceeds with the goal in mind—that opioid use is a means to accomplish improved function and quality of life—then I believe their use is justified.

When it comes to side effects, while it's true that opioids are notorious for causing constipation, this problem can be treated and even avoided if you adjust your diet (e.g., add more fiber and fresh fruits and vegetables; avoid processed, sugary foods; drink eight glasses of water daily) and regularly use laxatives and stool softeners. Although all opioid users do not become constipated, those who do typically require a daily stimulant laxative (e.g., senna) to maintain regularity. It is very important that such patients take a laxative regularly rather than as needed.

Based on the results of several studies and personal experience, the most serious risk posed by opioids is compromised mobility and falls, often with associated hip and other fractures. This is primarily a concern among older patients, while among younger patients, a different compromised ability— daytime drowsiness and cognitive problems—can be a challenge, especially as these symptoms can affect the ability to work, drive, and care for one's family.

Before I prescribe an opioid for patients, I counsel them about potential side effects, including falls, fractures, mental fogginess, and drowsiness. If patients currently have ambulatory problems, I try to optimize their mobility before they start the drug by sending them for physical therapy and having them learn to use an assistive device, such as a cane or walker.

I think of Herbert, for example, who was sixty-eight when he came to see me. Herbert had been diagnosed with lumbar spinal stenosis when he was only forty years old. At that time, his doctor performed a laminectomy (see chapter 8), which relieved the pain enough so that he could continue his work at an automobile factory, where he remained for twenty-five years until he retired at age sixty-five. During those years, he had recurring pain, which he treated regularly with anti-inflammatory drugs and with epidural steroid injections on several occasions. The injections had provided temporary relief.

By the time Herbert's son, Chet, brought his father in to see me, it had been three years since Herbert's last injection series. Along with the back pain, Herbert had significant pain in his left leg, and he was favoring that side with the help of a cane. His pain, disability, and fear of leaving the house and possibly injuring himself kept him homebound and away from activities he had once enjoyed, including fishing and going to church and volunteering on its special events committee. Chet expressed concern about not only his father's lack of mobility but also his deepening depression and social isolation.

Over the years, Herbert had been taking several NSAIDs, but by the time he came to see me, he was taking only naproxen twice a day and an antidepressant, amitriptyline (Elavil), once a day. After a thorough examination, I prescribed physical therapy and cognitive-behavioral therapy and changed his medications. In this case, I believed an opioid (controlled-release oxycodone), given for the short term, was appropriate, until Herbert could learn good coping skills through cognitive-behavioral therapy. I also discontinued the amitriptyline and substituted the SSRI citalopram (Celexa), because I believed it would be more effective against his depression and because it is associated with milder side effects. Within two months, Herbert said his pain was more than 50 percent better, he was no longer depressed, and he was actively involved with his church once again.

How Opioids Work

Opioids relieve pain in two ways. First, they attach to specific proteins, called opioid receptors, on the surface of cells in the brain, spinal cord, and gastrointestinal tract and stop the transmission of pain signals to the brain. Second, they change the perception of pain in the brain. How well an opioid relieves symptoms and the effects it has on pain depend on the dose you take, the form of the drug (oral, intravenous, intramuscular, rectal), your physical and emotional state, any past experiences you've had with the drug, and other medications you may be taking at the time. You may also develop a tolerance to opioids or even a cross-tolerance, which means long-term use of one opioid may cause you to develop a tolerance to other opioids. I want to point out here that the notion of tolerance is not a black-and-white issue. It can be difficult to distinguish between experiencing a diminished benefit from a drug because you have developed a tolerance to it or because the pain or other condition you are treating is getting worse.

Opioid Overview

Here are the more common opioids, with a few of the available brand names, your physician may prescribe. All are available in oral forms, and one (fentanyl) is also available in a transdermal patch.

- **Morphine** (MS Contin, Avinza). A natural opioid (derived from poppies, thus technically called an opiate) and the one often referred to as the "gold standard" of opioids, as it is the one against which all other opioids are compared.

- **Codeine** (generic only). Another natural opioid (i.e., an opiate), it is usually prescribed for pain that is less severe than that treated with morphine. Codeine is an ingredient in many cough syrups and is the "other" active ingredient in Tylenol #2, #3, and #4.
- **Hydrocodone** (Lorcet, Lortab, Norco, Vicodin; all also contain acetaminophen). Hydrocodone is a semisynthetic opioid that is often combined with a nonopioid painkiller; in this case, acetaminophen. The acetaminophen enhances the effects of hydrocodone and has the added benefit of reducing fever.
- **Oxycodone** (OxyContin, Percolone, Roxicodone; combined with acetaminophen in Percocet, Endocet). Oxycodone is a semisynthetic opioid that is often used alone or along with acetaminophen or aspirin. The addition of acetaminophen or aspirin enhances the effects of oxycodone and has the added benefit of reducing fever.
- **Hydromorphone** (Dilaudid). Another semisynthetic opioid that is often used in older adults and in patients who have renal failure.
- **Fentanyl** (Actiq, Duragesic [transdermal]). This synthetic opioid is available in an oral form as well as a transdermal patch, which generally has fewer side effects than oral opioids, as well as the lowest potential for abuse among drugs in this class. Research shows that transdermal fentanyl significantly decreased pain and improved functioning in patients with chronic low back pain. In one study of sixty-four patients who had back pain associated with vertebral osteoporosis, treatment with transdermal fentanyl for four weeks resulted in a significant improvement in the ability to undergo physical therapy and a significant improvement in the quality of life.

- **Tramadol** (Ultram). A synthetic medication with opioid properties, it is often used in patients who have high blood pressure, congestive heart failure, or renal insufficiency.
- **Propoxyphene** (Darvon). Another synthetic opioid, it has never been shown to be superior to placebo in relieving pain, so it can cause many of the side effects of the effective opioids but none of the benefits.
- **Meperidine** (Demerol). A synthetic opioid that has a higher incidence of side effects than some others.
- **Methadone** (Dolophine). Although many people think of this drug as one used to help individuals who were addicted to opioids avoid withdrawal symptoms, it is also used to treat severe pain. Patient response is mixed, with some finding the side effects intolerable but others very pleased with the results.

Other Caveats

In addition to constipation, drowsiness, and dizziness or light-headedness, other potential side effects of opioid use include euphoria, nausea, vomiting, respiratory depression, dilated pupils, and sweating. Opioids should be used with extreme caution if you have asthma or other respiratory problems and should not be taken without first consulting your doctor if you have seizures; any type of brain disorder; head injury; lung disease; prostate problems; urinary difficulties; gallstones; colitis; a history of alcohol or drug abuse; or heart, liver, kidney, or thyroid disease.

If you have been taking opioids and want to stop, don't do it abruptly. Symptoms of withdrawal may begin as quickly as a few hours after you dramatically reduce your dose, and symptoms may peak two to three days later. To prevent withdrawal symptoms, allow your physician to help you taper off the drug(s) gradually. Symptoms of withdrawal include craving for the drug, moodiness, insomnia, yawning, abdominal cramps, diarrhea, and restlessness.

Opioids also need to be used with caution when taken with other drugs. Alcohol, sleeping pills, tranquilizers, and other medications that have an impact on the central nervous system should not be taken along with opioids, because the combination can result in serious consequences. The same is true of drugs that reduce blood pressure (e.g., beta-blockers, antihypertensives), as the combination may result in abnormally low blood pressure. Use of cimetidine (Tagamet) along with opioids may result in breathing problems, disorientation, seizures, and confusion. Herbs that produce a sedative effect also may cause potentially dangerous depressant reactions if used along with opioids. Some of those herbs include calendula, capsicum, catnip, goldenseal, gotu kola, hops, kava, passionflower, sage, Siberian ginseng, skullcap, St. John's wort, and valerian, among others.

I want to add yet another word of caution to older adults who take opioids. As with the tricyclic antidepressants, side effects such as falls and constipation may impose a greater risk in older patients than in younger patients. Thus, these medications should be used carefully, and older adults who take them should be monitored closely by a physician.

IN CONCLUSION . . .

I have a love-hate relationship with pain medications. I am thankful they are available for those patients who cannot get through a day without them. And I am saddened by the fact that far too many patients continue to take them and become controlled by them and their side effects. I quietly celebrate whenever one of my patients successfully divests himself or herself of pain medication, because it means he or she has reached a new milestone of independence and freedom. Often, the first step toward such freedom is knowledge. If you are taking a pain medication that is discussed in this chapter or any other painkiller and you want to move to a less toxic drug or away from drugs altogether, talk to your physician to learn about the options available to you.

Chapter 8

Step 6: Surgery and Other
Invasive Treatments

Occasionally, when patients have tried conventional and alternative approaches to manage and treat their chronic back pain and all of the options have failed to provide adequate pain relief or improved quality of life, more dramatic measures may be necessary, be it a surgical intervention or the implantation of devices that can deliver pain relief. I think it's fair to say that *95 percent of patients with chronic low back pain should view surgery solely as an elective procedure, to be contemplated only after first methodically trying as many nonsurgical options as is feasible*, like those discussed throughout this book. The remaining 5 percent, which includes patients who experience a sudden worsening of symptoms associated with serious neurological compromise, such as loss of bladder or bowel control, should proceed to surgery before further damage occurs.

I can only assume that if you are reading this chapter, you

are contemplating back surgery for yourself or a loved one. While I am not glad you are thinking about such a step, I am happy you are investigating your options. One piece of information you should know is that, according to a study released in June 2005 in the international journal *Spine*, most surgeons are "overly optimistic" when they talk to their patients about the probable outcome of their back surgery. In fact, in one recent study, nearly 40 percent of 197 back surgery patients surveyed experienced no measurable reduction in pain after their surgery, even though their doctors had predicted a "great improvement." This high percentage of unsatisfied patients occurs for a number of reasons, not least of which are that some doctors simply routinely recommend surgery without adequately considering alternatives, while some patients are desperate and ask for surgery because they believe it's their last hope.

Before you opt for surgery, I recommend you thoroughly review the measures you've taken thus far, consider those you have not tried, learn all you can about the surgical and invasive procedures available, and consult with your health-care providers. As a starting point, in this chapter, we look at some of the more common invasive procedures performed for chronic back pain, the reason they may be done, risks and benefits, and guidelines on how to help you recover from each of these procedures.

I also discuss a phenomenon called failed back surgery syndrome (FBSS) and why you need to know about it before you make a decision concerning whether to undergo back surgery. Related to this issue is another factor we need to mention. According to research data presented in February 2005 at the American Academy of Orthopaedic Surgeons in Washington, D.C., many patients who seek surgery for their chronic back pain have other health and social issues that not only affect their lives but can also have a major impact on their recovery from surgery. It has become clear that failure to recognize and manage these factors can have considerable negative consequences on your quality of life; thus, I include them in our discussion, so you will be able to make a more informed decision about back surgery.

IS SURGERY THE RIGHT DECISION FOR YOU?

"I felt like my life was over," said Robert, a fifty-five-year-old self-employed electrician who had been suffering with chronic low back pain for nearly a year. "I couldn't work, I couldn't take care of my family, and I didn't even want to get up in the morning anymore. Exercises, acupuncture, epidural injections—nothing worked. I was taking narcotics to help me get through each day, but the side effects were too much. I was hoping surgery would be the answer, the end of my pain. I felt it was my last chance for anything resembling a normal life."

Making a decision about whether to undergo back surgery is a challenge. For one thing, you are under stress and in pain, conditions that are not best for making decisions. For another, there are many factors to consider and medical terms to grapple with, both of which only add to the stress. Many patients are like Robert; they hope, even believe, that surgery will be *the* answer. And for some patients it is.

But for far too many others, surgery is not the right decision. Here are a few things to consider.

- If you think back or spine surgery is going to "fix" you and that no further treatment will be necessary, think again. Often, continued therapies and rehabilitation are necessary if you expect success after back surgery.

- In many cases, back surgery is necessary to provide enough pain relief so you can begin rehabilitation, but the surgery should be viewed as only one factor in your healing process.

- One very important thing to think about if you are considering back or spine surgery is a phenomenon called failed back surgery syndrome. This is not a syndrome at all, but a generalized term used to describe the condition of patients who undergo surgery of the back or spine and who do not get a satisfactory result. The number of patients who fall into this category is 30 percent or greater. I explain this phenomenon in more depth later in this chapter (see Failed Back Surgery Syndrome).

- The failure of nonsurgical treatments to relieve your pain is not enough to support a decision to have spine surgery—there must be a clear-cut, physical cause of your pain. In addition, the anatomic cause should be identifiable (e.g., on an MRI scan, CT scan, myelogram, or discogram), and the abnormality identified on imaging should clearly explain your symptoms. (For example, if imaging shows an abnormality on the left side of your spine but your pain is on the right, another cause for your pain should be sought.)

To help you make a decision about back surgery and to select a surgeon, I have provided a list of questions you can ask yourself and the likely candidates.

GUIDELINES TO CONSIDER WHEN CONTEMPLATING BACK SURGERY

Questions to ask your doctor about your condition and possible procedures:

- What specific physical condition do I have that would be addressed by surgery?
- What would happen if I choose not to have surgery?
- What alternatives do I have to surgery, and how effective are they in addressing my condition?
- What specific procedure(s) is (are) recommended for my condition?
- What are the risks associated with the procedure(s)?
- What is the typical success rate (e.g., percentage of pain relief, improvement in function, and so on) of this procedure in individuals similar in age, condition, and accompanying medical issues?
- Can I speak with other patients who have undergone a similar procedure?
- How is (are) the procedure(s) done?
- How long will I be in the hospital?
- What is the recovery time (i.e., how long until a return to normal functioning)?
- What type of postsurgical therapy will I need?
- What type of permanent limitations can I expect after surgery?
- What happens if the surgery fails? What are my options?

Questions about the surgeon:

- How many of the recommended procedures does the surgeon do yearly?

- What special training does the surgeon have? (This is especially important in spinal fusion cases.)

- Does the surgeon seem genuinely interested in you; that is, does he or she ask questions about factors that could have a significant impact on your recovery, such as your expectations of the surgery, amount of stress in your life, concerns about work or returning to work, ability to participate in social activities and hobbies, level of family support, and so on?

You should look for another surgeon if he or she:

- Discourages or feels threatened because you have sought or are about to seek a second opinion. (NOTE: *always* get a second opinion.)

- Tries to scare you into making a quick decision or is heavy-handed in how he or she presents information about surgery. If you feel uncomfortable with any surgeon, that's a good indication to look for another physician.

- Claims he or she can guarantee you'll be pain-free or can cure you. You may *want* to hear those words, but they may not be realistic.

- Suggests you undergo exploratory surgery. Back surgery should not be done unless there is concrete evidence (from imaging) of a physical abnormality.

- Disregards or downplays other conservative treatment options, including injection therapy, medication (both oral and implanted), and stimulation therapy.

Are Your Expectations Realistic?

Back or spine surgery should be recognized for what it is: an attempt, regardless of what the procedure is, to modify anatomy in one of two general ways: it can decompress the nerve root(s) or spinal cord that is (are) being pinched or stabilize a painful joint. If one or both of these conditions is causing you to have chronic back pain and one or both is corrected surgically, then you may enjoy pain relief. But although pain relief is usually the chief goal, an improvement in function is also important to many patients. In fact, because total pain relief after surgery is rare, it is often best for patients to think about how important improved functioning is compared with pain relief.

But how much pain relief can you expect from surgery? Is there more than one type of surgery that could provide good results? These are questions you need to ask and discuss with your primary-care physician and a surgeon.

The decision of whether or not to undergo back surgery for low back pain is nearly always yours. You should not be pressured, scared, or rushed into making a quick decision. In fact, situations that require immediate, emergency surgery are rare. They may include

- cauda equina syndrome, characterized by sudden bowel and/or bladder incontinence or progressive weakness in the legs.
- abdominal aortic aneurysm that either ruptures or one in which blood leaks along the walls of the aorta (known as an aortic dissection). These types of aneurysms are characterized by severe and continuous pain in the abdomen and back that comes on suddenly.

In the absence of an emergency, you should take the time you need to learn all you can about any proposed surgical or other invasive procedure before you make a decision to proceed. I suggest you collect information from several sources, including your primary-care physician, a spine surgeon, other patients who have had the procedure you are contemplating, and the great amount of literature on the topic that is available in books, on the Internet, in consumer and medical libraries, and from various organizations (see the suggested reading and videos/DVDs section).

You should know, for example, the usual success rate for the type of surgery you are considering. For instance, a discectomy or microdiscectomy, when performed to correct a herniated lumbar disc that is causing leg pain, is highly predictable. The same procedures done to relieve lower back pain without leg pain is more likely to fail. The main reason back surgery fails to relieve pain is that health-care practitioners do not accurately identify the cause of the pain (including missing a cause when there is more than one), and so the area operated on is not the source of the pain. This is not the only reason back surgeries fail, however. I discuss other reasons in the Failed Back Surgery Syndrome section below.

Open or Minimally Invasive?

If you meet the criteria for surgery, you may also be allowed to choose the procedure. Spinal surgeries can be either open or minimally invasive. Open procedures require larger incisions; more anesthesia; and longer operating, hospitalization, and recovery times. Minimally invasive techniques involve tiny incisions through which surgeons can insert small, specialized instruments, such as an endoscope, which allow them to see a lighted, magnified view of the surgical site. In some cases, lasers may be used to eliminate or separate tissues. With the help of computer-assisted image guidance, surgeons can use specially designed instruments to implant necessary hardware, such as screws and rods to stabilize the spine. This type of computer-assisted surgery is not yet widely available but will be as more surgeons become familiar with the technique.

The goals of minimally invasive procedures are to achieve more rapid recovery, reduce postoperative pain and the risk of infection, and leave much less conspicuous scars. Although it seems obvious to choose a minimally invasive procedure, not all neurosurgeons are specially trained to perform these procedures, and not all hospitals have the special equipment that is needed. Both of these limitations are expected to improve in the near future (see the epilogue). You may also have a situation that requires open surgery. You need to discuss your options with your surgeon.

Will Patience Pay Off?

The most common surgical procedure performed in the lower back is removal of a herniated disc. Removal of a herniated disc is sometimes considered for patients who have not responded to epidural steroid injections and an exercise program (including dynamic stabilization exercises and the McKenzie Method). However, studies show that most herniated discs, even large ones, disappear within one year without surgery. Thus, you may be able to avoid surgery and possible post-surgical complications if you are patient and continue using other treatments while giving the disc time to heal. For patients who do choose surgery, there are several surgical techniques used to deal with a herniated disc. These and other surgical procedures are discussed in this chapter.

After Back Surgery

Postsurgical care is different for each type of back or spine surgery performed. Some procedures allow you to return to your normal activities within a day or two; others require you to carefully monitor your movements for weeks or months. Therefore, I have included postsurgical guidelines as part of the discussions of the individual procedures.

Generally, before you leave the hospital, you should meet with a physical therapist or consult with a health-care professional who can show you how to feel safe and comfortable when performing such activities as climbing stairs, sitting, and getting into and out of a car or bed. If you do not already have a physical therapy program, your physician may prescribe one for your specific condition for you to do at home. In most cases, daily walks are encouraged to hasten the healing process and reduce the risk of scar tissue forming, with other levels of activity dependent on the surgery performed and your physical condition.

LAMINECTOMY AND LAMINOTOMY

For some people who have a herniated disc, spinal stenosis, or spinal tumors that have not responded to other treatments, a laminectomy or laminotomy could be a viable option. A lumbar laminectomy involves removal of the entire lamina (the small, bony plate located in the back of each vertebra), while a laminotomy is partial removal. The goal of these procedures is to widen the spinal canal and thus relieve pressure on the spinal cord or spinal nerve. A discectomy or microdiscectomy is often also performed at the same time (see below).

A laminectomy or laminotomy may be performed either as

an open or minimally invasive procedure. Generally, the surgeon makes an incision in the lower back and locates the compressed nerve. At this point, some or all of the lamina may be removed, along with associated ligament. In many cases the nerve compression is caused by a herniated disc, but other causes may include a disc fragment, a bone spur, a protruding or degenerated disc, or a cyst or tumor. The surgeon removes the source of the compression and, if necessary, may fuse vertebrae and use metal screws or rods to help support the spine and provide stability (see Spinal Fusion). The incision is then closed, and the procedure is complete. The surgery usually takes one to three hours, depending on whether any spine support is inserted.

Pain medication, either oral or intravenous, is given post-surgery. Once you leave the recovery room and are in a hospital room, you will be encouraged to walk within hours of the procedure. To protect your back from pain and injury post-surgery, a nurse or therapist will review some guidelines with you. Here are a few of what you can expect.

- Stand up straight and keep your shoulders and hips in a straight line. Tighten your abdominal muscles to help support your spine.
- When you bend, do so at the hips, not at the waist. Do not twist at the shoulders or hips.
- To get into bed, back up to the edge of the bed, tighten your abdominal muscles, and lower yourself using your legs. Once you are seated, use your arms to lower your body onto the bed as you lift your feet into the bed. Then roll your body as one unit onto your back. Do not twist your shoulders or hips.
- The recommended sleeping positions may be different

from what you are used to, but you do have a choice: you can lie on your back and place pillows under your knees and neck, or lie on one side with your knees slightly bent and a pillow between your knees to keep them a comfortable, natural distance apart.

• To get out of bed, tighten your abdominal muscles and roll onto your side as a unit. Scoot to the edge of the bed and use your arms to raise your body. As you raise your body, slowly swing your legs to the floor. Place one foot behind the other, tighten your abdominal muscles, and use your legs to raise your body from the bed.

Most patients can go home within hours of undergoing a minimally invasive laminectomy, while an overnight stay or two is usual after an open procedure. Recovery is similar: just a few days for a minimally invasive procedure, and a few weeks for an open one. In both situations, your doctor or therapist should have you return to physical therapy and your exercise program, including frequent walks, within days.

DISCECTOMY AND MICRODISCECTOMY

Both of these terms refer to the surgical removal of a small segment of the bone over the nerve root and/or part or all of an intervertebral disc from under the nerve root. These surgeries are usually performed for a lumbar herniated disc that is accompanied by leg or buttocks pain or weakness that is severe, disabling, and/or persistent (for at least six weeks) that has not responded to nonsurgical treatment. The difference between the two procedures is that in an open discectomy, the surgeon makes an incision that allows him or her to directly visualize the herniated disc in order to remove it. In a microdiscectomy, the surgeon uses a camera to visualize the affected disc, micro-surgical techniques, and very small incisions (one to one and a half inches), which reduces recovery time and the risk of complications. In some cases, general anesthesia is not required for a microdiscectomy. Both of these surgical procedures are frequently performed along with a laminectomy or laminotomy.

Usually, discectomy and microdiscectomy are done on an outpatient basis, although sometimes one overnight hospital stay is recommended. Because the procedures don't require the surgeon to make any mechanical changes to your back, you can expect to return to normal functioning immediately after microdiscectomy or a few days after discectomy (because of the longer incision). The best medicine after microdiscectomy and discectomy is an exercise program that includes strengthening, stretching, and aerobic conditioning to help prevent the recurrence of disc herniation and back pain.

Leonard's Story

A daily exercise program, including long walks, was part of Leonard's routine following his microdiscectomy. Leonard is a seventy-one-year-old retired civil engineer who had started out thoroughly enjoying his retirement with his wife of fifty years. Together they regularly took road trips from Pittsburgh to visit their three children in Chicago, Minneapolis, and Las Vegas and were active in their church. Leonard spent much time doing wood carving and taking daily walks around the lake. After undergoing emergency heart surgery in June 2003, from which he recovered well, he was diagnosed with polymyalgia rheumatica (a type of arthritis that causes muscles, typically in the neck, lower back, hips, and thighs, to become very sore, stiff, and inflamed, but does not affect the joints). His doctor at the time prescribed prednisone, a steroid, and he soon felt better.

In July 2004, Leonard began to experience sharp lower back pain during a road trip from Pittsburgh to Minneapolis. The pain started on the left lower back and buttocks and radiated down the back of his thigh and the side of his leg to his ankle. Over the next few months, the pain improved on the left side, and Leonard continued his daily walks and even went ice skating in November of that year. But by late December 2004, the pain recurred in his lower back and buttocks and appeared in his right leg. He was very fatigued, and walking and standing had become increasingly difficult. The only time he got relief, he said, was when he was sitting or lying in a curled-up position. His physician sent him for an MRI in early January 2005, which showed degenerative disc disease at several levels in his lower back. When the doctor recommended surgery, Leonard said he wanted a second opinion.

Leonard came to see me shortly after he had the MRI. His walk was guarded, and when he stood, he was flexed forward. When I did the physical examination, I noted that he had scoliosis as well as tenderness over both sacroiliac joints, the right piriformis, and the right tensor fascia lata. I gave Leonard my diagnosis—sciatica associated with scoliosis, myofascial pain, and sacroiliac joint syndrome—and recommended he immediately undergo epidural corticosteroid injections and physical therapy to relieve his pain. I also suggested he begin a series of PENS treatments and gave him a prescription for a mild opioid (Vicodin) to take as needed to help him through this aggressive treatment campaign.

Leonard was up for the fight, and he followed through on all the recommendations. "I have too many things I want to do," he said, "and I can't let this get me down." Yet despite all his efforts and dedication, his condition continued to worsen over the next six weeks, and he became very discouraged. At this point we discussed surgery, and I referred him to a neurosurgeon, who performed a microdiscectomy. He underwent the outpatient procedure on a Tuesday and was back doing light stretching and strengthening exercises by Thursday, along with short daily walks. Within four months of surgery, he and his wife were on another road trip, and he had returned to his long daily walks and wood carving. He says he has some intermittent, minimal pain, which he treats with ibuprofen as needed (he does not need the Vicodin) and continues to do daily stretching exercises and strengthening exercises several times a week.

Postsurgery

Eighty to 90 percent of patients who undergo a discectomy or microdiscectomy have good results, although individuals who have pain in the legs generally experience more pain relief than those who have the procedure to relieve low back pain alone. It can take several weeks to months for the nerve root to heal completely and for any numbness or weakness to improve, although most patients feel some relief immediately after surgery.

Possible complications from open discectomy include risk of infection, bleeding, leakage of cerebrospinal fluid (which occurs in 1 to 2 percent of these surgeries), injury to the arteries and veins near the spine, bowel or bladder incontinence, or injury to the nerve tissue. If you do experience a leak of cerebrospinal fluid, your doctor will instruct you to lie flat in bed for one to two days to allow the leak to seal. Such leakage does not change the results of the surgery.

In 5 to 10 percent of open discectomy cases, disc herniation recurs in the same disc. Although it can happen at any time, it is most likely to occur within the first three months after surgery. Infrequently, a patient has multiple herniated disc recurrences, and in such instances spinal fusion is often recommended.

SPINAL FUSION

Many surgeons consider spinal fusion to be the surgery of choice for just about any type of mechanical low back pain, including pain caused by a degenerated disc, spinal stenosis, vertebral fractures, spondylolisthesis, tumors, and scoliosis. For spinal fusion to be successful, the exact cause of your pain must be identified, which typically means you must undergo the standard history taking; complete physical examination, including comprehensive musculoskeletal and neurological examinations; X-rays; an MRI; and additional scans as needed until the cause of your pain is definitively found.

What Is Spinal Fusion?

The goal of spinal fusion is to obtain a solid union between two or more vertebrae and to stop the movement in the segment of the spine that is causing pain. To achieve this, a surgeon grafts a small piece of bone, usually taken from the patient's pelvis but occasionally from a bone bank, onto the spine to stimulate the vertebrae to fuse together. Depending on how stable the spine is, the surgeon may or may not also implant metal screws, cages, plates, or rods to help support the spine and make it more stable. A spinal fusion can be performed either from the back (posterior approach), from the front (anterior approach), or a combination of both. When the lower back is involved, the surgery is usually performed from the back.

The success rate for spinal fusion is about 80 percent, which means 80 percent of patients achieve some pain relief and improvement in functioning. Twenty percent of patients do not improve.

What Happens After Surgery?

Spinal fusion is a more complex procedure than, say, a laminectomy or discectomy, and so postsurgery discomfort and recovery time are usually greater than with other types of spinal surgeries. (If you get a bone graft from your own pelvis, the discomfort is greater, because harvesting the graft involves surgery as well, so you have two surgical sites that must heal.) To help control the pain, your physician may prescribe a patient-controlled pain-control pump, which allows you to deliver a predetermined amount of a narcotic through an intravenous line when you need it. The hospital stay after spinal fusion is generally three or four days or even longer, compared with an overnight stay after a laminectomy or discectomy.

It will also take longer for you to return to your presurgery level of activity, because the bone needs to heal. In fact, it typically takes at least six weeks for bone healing to be evident on X-ray, and during that time, your activities will be very restricted. After that time, you will be able to increase your activities, as more significant healing occurs at three to four months postsurgery. Many patients are surprised to learn that it can take up to two years for healing and bone remodeling to be completed.

For some spinal fusion patients, the recovery process includes the temporary use of a brace to provide support and comfort and/or to limit motion. Recovery should always include a rehabilitation program that may include strengthening exercises, aerobic conditioning, and any specially designed exercises that will help you at work or at home.

If you hope to return to work after a spinal fusion, how quickly that occurs will depend on the extent of the surgery, the type of work you do, and if you have any other medical conditions. If, for example, you are young and otherwise healthy and have a sedentary job and you've undergone a posterior fusion, you may be able to return to work within six weeks. If you are older, have a physically demanding job, and/or the fusion involved more than two vertebrae, you may be out of work for six months or longer.

If you smoke and have spinal fusion surgery, know that nicotine can inhibit healing of the bone. One study shows that failure of the bone to fuse is lowest in nonsmokers (14 percent), slightly higher in patients who quit smoking for at least six months after surgery (17 percent), and highest for patients who still smoked (26 percent).

What's the usual long-term outcome of spinal fusion surgery? Eighteen months after her surgery, fifty-one-year-old Claudia noted, "Before surgery, I was operating at about 25 percent; now I'm at about 75 percent. My back will never be normal, and I have to avoid certain repetitive, strenuous activities that involve lifting or twisting. So I don't shovel snow or rake leaves, which doesn't break my heart. But I have much less pain than I used to, and I can do most activities in moderation. And that's a big improvement."

The good news about a spinal fusion is that once it heals, it rarely breaks down. It does, however, place additional stress on the vertebrae adjacent to the fusion site, which can speed up the degeneration of these areas. To help prevent this deterioration, it is best to avoid the types of activities Claudia mentioned.

VERTEBROPLASTY AND KYPHOPLASTY

Vertebroplasty and kyphoplasty are two relatively new and related procedures that are used to treat chronic low back pain associated with osteoporotic compression fractures, painful vertebrae due to metastases, vertebral hemangiomas (abnormal accumulation of blood vessels in the vertebrae), multiple myeloma (cancer of the bone marrow), and similar conditions.

An estimated 700,000 vertebral body compression fractures occur in the United States each year, and virtually all of them are associated with osteoporosis and lead to progressive deformity. About one-third of them cause chronic back pain. Vertebroplasty or kyphoplasty may be recommended in some cases, not only to relieve the pain but to strengthen and stabilize the spine and thus help prevent further damage and permanent disability. The advantage of kyphoplasty over vertebroplasty is that the former has the ability to restore height to the spine, which helps reduce the risk of deformity.

Vertebroplasty

Vertebroplasty (which literally means "fixing the vertebral body") involves injection of polymethylmethacrylate (PMMA), a type of bone cement, into the vertebral body at the site of the compression fracture. Once the thick paste has been injected, it hardens quickly and helps strengthen and stabilize the vertebral body and thus helps relieve pain.

The procedure is done under local or general anesthesia. Once the surgical site has been prepared, the surgeon slowly inserts a special bone needle into your back. A fluoroscope or CT is used to help the surgeon guide the path of the needle. When the needle is in place, a small amount of PMMA is injected into the vertebral body, usually on both the left and right sides. Often the cement is mixed with an antibiotic to reduce the risk of infection.

After the vertebroplasty, you will need to lie still for several hours in a recovery room; then you will be allowed to go home. Your discharge instructions may include the following guidelines:

- Take any pain medications as directed.
- Wear your back brace, if one has been prescribed.
- Do not bathe or shower for twenty-four hours.
- Avoid any heavy lifting (nothing more than 1 pound) for three months.
- Continue with (or begin) a walking program.
- Schedule a visit with your physician for six weeks post-surgery.
- Alert your physician if you experience fever, chills, redness, or drainage from your incision. (A slight amount of drainage is normal during the first twenty-four to forty-eight hours after surgery.)

Kyphoplasty

Kyphoplasty is a variation of a vertebroplasty and is a bit more complex, because it involves insertion of a balloon catheter into the collapsed fractured vertebral body before the PMMA is injected. Once the surgical site has been prepared, the surgeon makes two small incisions (approximately 1 centimeter each) and uses CT or fluoroscopy to help guide a probe that is placed into the vertebral space where the fracture is located. The bone is drilled, and a balloon is inserted and inflated to the desired height. The balloon is then removed, and the PMMA is injected.

After surgery, you can expect to be up and walking around within a few hours and then be discharged within twenty-four hours. Within two weeks, you should be able to begin (or continue with) physical therapy and strengthening exercises. Also within that same two-week period, if you are like the vast majority of patients, you should experience 80 to 90 percent pain relief.

That certainly was true for Walter, a sixty-year-old retired bank executive who had been taking corticosteroids for many years to treat a chronic lung condition. The drugs took their toll on his bones, and he developed osteoporosis. One day he bent down to pick up the newspaper from the driveway and felt a piercing pain in his back. He was diagnosed with a compression fracture and experienced debilitating chronic back pain that he began treating with opioids. After several weeks, however, he decided to undergo kyphoplasty, and once the procedure was done, he was nearly free of back pain and no longer needed the opioids.

What to Expect from Vertebroplasty and Kyphoplasty

Both vertebroplasty and kyphoplasty have good success and satisfaction rates. In one study conducted at the Mayo Clinic (Cleveland), thirty patients (twenty-four with osteoporotic compression fractures and six with compression fractures due to multiple myeloma) underwent seventy kyphoplasty procedures and reported significant improvement in pain and function, as well as partial restoration of height in 70 percent of the vertebral bodies. In another study, 63 percent of patients reported complete pain relief, and 32 percent said pain relief was moderate after vertebroplasty.

How long can you expect to have pain relief following these surgeries? The results vary. Many patients say they still have significant relief five years after surgery, although others experience a recurrence of moderate to severe pain sooner.

Vertebroplasty and kyphoplasty are not without complications. Vertebroplasty requires that the PMMA be injected under high pressure, which can lead to leaks of small amounts of the cement, although it usually does not cause a significant problem. Between 4 and 6 percent of vertebroplasty patients have serious complications, including rib fractures, infection, and neuritis (inflamed nerves). New compression fractures also may develop adjacent to fractures treated previously.

Kyphoplasty has a much lower risk of cement leakage because the cement can be injected under lower pressure. The risk of significant infection, bleeding, nerve injury, paralysis, and pulmonary embolism is less than 1 percent for each. Between 10 and 15 percent of kyphoplasty patients experience an additional compression fracture at other vertebrae. It appears that these fractures are a result of having weak bones because of osteoporosis and not a result of the surgery itself.

IMPLANTABLE SPINAL NEUROSTIMULATOR

For patients who have chronic nerve pain that does not respond to other therapeutic approaches, a surgically implanted spinal cord stimulator may be the answer. This approach is also known as neuromodulation. The device delivers electrical impulses to the spinal cord via epidural electrodes, which stimulate the body's pain inhibitory systems and block incoming pain signals. Use of a spinal cord stimulator is usually reserved for patients who have chronic nerve pain that has not responded to other treatments and that radiates to the extremities and those who have failed back surgery syndrome (FBSS).

Studies of patients with FBSS who opted for the implant show that more than half of the patients reported greater than 50 percent pain relief up to several years after the procedure was done, and 47 percent reported greater than 50 percent relief five years after implantation. The patients also reported greater independence, a better quality of life, reduced hospitalizations, and lower related health-care costs. In one study, researchers found that the implantable device improved functional capacity 61 percent and reduced the use of pain medication by 90 percent during a four-year follow-up. Pain relief can last as long as twenty years after the device is implanted.

Although serious side effects are rare, some patients experience shocking sensations or jolts that require the surgeon to make adjustments to the device. Patients who have an implantable cardiac pacemaker or defibrillator or who are likely to undergo MRI regularly are not candidates for a neurostimulator. Generally, anyone who has an implantable spinal neurostimulator should wear a medical alert identifier in case they are in an emergency situation, as medical personnel should know this information.

INTRASPINAL DRUG-INFUSION PUMP

An intraspinal drug-infusion pump delivers pain medication (usually morphine) directly to the space around the spinal cord. Because the morphine is delivered directly to the spine and does not have to be processed through the gastrointestinal tract, an implantable spinal pump allows you to use a much lower dose of morphine to control pain; in fact, about three hundred times less. This also means any side effects from the morphine are minimized, and the risk of addiction is virtually nil. Research shows that fewer than one in one thousand patients who take morphine through an intraspinal drug-infusion system become addicted to the drug.

Use of an intraspinal drug-infusion pump is usually reserved for individuals whose chronic pain responds to oral medications but the medication dose required is quite high and is associated with intolerable side effects.

The pump is a round metal disk about one inch thick and three inches in diameter that is surgically implanted just underneath the skin, usually in the lower abdomen. The medication is added to the pump periodically (usually monthly) by a physician, who injects it through the skin into a reservoir in the device, and it is delivered to the spinal canal through a catheter.

Although this method of pain relief was originally used mainly by cancer patients, it is now frequently prescribed to manage nonmalignant chronic pain, including low back pain. Studies show that 60 to 81 percent of patients with persistent nonmalignant pain who used the pump rated their pain relief as good to excellent. In addition to better pain control, patients have also reported improved function, enhanced quality of life, and a reduced need to take other painkillers.

Intraspinal drug-infusion pumps do have a downside, although problems are uncommon. Mechanical difficulties, such as a broken, dislodged, blocked, or kinked catheter, may occur. Because the pump is inserted surgically, there is always a risk, albeit small, of infection. On rare occasions, inflammation may develop at the site of the catheter tip. This reaction is more likely to occur in people who use the pump long term. Indications that inflammation may be present include a progressive change in the intensity, character, or quality of pain; numbness or tingling; bowel and/or bladder changes; gait disturbances; paralysis; and drug withdrawal symptoms.

FAILED BACK SURGERY SYNDROME

When was the last time you heard someone talk about "failed hip surgery syndrome," "failed knee surgery syndrome," or "failed hernia surgery syndrome"? You haven't, because the failure rates for these and many other surgical procedures are relatively low. The same cannot be said about back surgery. According to the American Academy of Orthopaedic Surgeons, for example, 20 to 30 percent of the more than 200,000 laminectomies performed every year are unsuccessful.

Back surgery often fails to provide the type of relief patients expect. When a discectomy, microdiscectomy, or laminectomy is performed for a compressed nerve in the lumbar spine and improvement occurs within three months of the surgery, improvement should continue. If, however, pain and related symptoms do not improve during those first three months, the surgery is considered to be unsuccessful, or failed. Patients who continue to have pain after surgery even after they have allowed enough time for healing to occur are then faced with the prospect of another surgery or ending up in a situation that may be worse than the one they were in before the surgery. These are possibilities you need to think about and discuss with your physician if you are considering back surgery.

Causes of Failed Back Surgery Syndrome

The term failed back surgery syndrome is a general phrase that describes a condition in which patients who have undergone back surgery have little or no relief postsurgery. As I mentioned previously, one criterion for back surgery is the presence of a physical, identifiable cause of the pain. After that, you choose the type of surgery that has a high degree of success with the specific cause of your pain. Even if these critically important factors are met, however, other potential causes for failure exist. For example,

- in cases of spinal fusion, sometimes the fusion fails or the bone implant fails. It takes at least three months for a solid fusion to take hold, and it often takes as long as one year. For this reason, most surgeons will not do a repeat back surgery for at least twelve months. Imaging of the spine often does not tell physicians whether the fusion has occurred, so if you have had spinal fusion and are still experiencing pain, there may be no way to know whether the fusion has "taken."

- the hardware (e.g., screws, rods) used in a spinal fusion may fail, especially if you have a very unstable spine. If surgery is done to help stabilize a highly unstable spine, it becomes a test of time: will the spine fuse and become stable first, or will the hardware fail first under the pressure? The risk of hardware failure increases the larger a patient is and the more vertebrae that are fused.

- in cases of lumbar decompression surgery for herniated discs or stenosis, there can be nerve damage that occurs during surgery, a nerve that does not heal after surgery, or the decompression itself could be inadequate.

- pain may return many years after a spinal fusion if a vertebra above the successfully fused one deteriorates.

- years after a lumbar laminectomy is done for spinal stenosis, the stenosis can return at the same location or at a different level of the spine.

- about 5 to 10 percent of patients who undergo lumbar laminectomy for disc herniation experience a recurrent herniation, usually within the first three months after surgery.

- on rare occasions, a surgeon does not see a bone fragment that is pinching a nerve and the patient continues to experience pain.

- on rare occasions, surgery is done at the wrong level of the spine or nerve damage occurs during a discectomy or a lumbar decompression, which has been reported in about 0.1 percent of cases. Such damage can be permanent, and an electromyelogram should be done to see the damage and determine whether healing may occur.

- if surgery for spinal stenosis fails to completely unpinch (decompress) the nerve root or spinal cord, the pain will continue after surgery.

- inadequate and/or improper postsurgery rehabilitation is also a cause of FBSS. Generally, the more extensive the back surgery and the longer you had your symptoms, the longer and more difficult your postoperative rehabilitation will be.

- back surgery sometimes brings other back problems to the forefront. For example, Madelaine, a forty-eight-year-old real estate adjuster, underwent a lumbar laminectomy and discectomy for disc herniation, and she was pleased that the pain in her leg was relieved. However, she still suffered with buttocks pain from spasms in the piriformis muscle, and so she said she felt her surgery had been a failure. However, what she needed was a physical therapy program, including a home exercise plan, to address the spasms, as well as a way to strengthen her muscles to support the work of the surgery. Once these efforts were put into place, she began to experience less pain and better mobility.

Madelaine's case is a good example of why, after back surgery, it is critical for you to follow the rehabilitation program ordered by your doctor and to follow postsurgery guidelines concerning activity. If you continue to experience pain after surgery and after you have allowed enough time for healing and rehabilitation, then a new evaluation may be needed to see if you have a new problem or if the original problem was not dealt with adequately.

More Than an Operation

One of the biggest mistakes back surgeons can make is believing they are treating only a person's back, when in fact they are having an impact on an individual's entire physical, social, emotional, mental, and spiritual well-being. "Back pain . . . [is] flavored by cognitive and social factors," notes Stanley A. Herring, M.D., clinical professor and medical director of the Spine Center at the University of Washington, Seattle. At the 2005 American Academy of Orthopaedic Surgeons meeting in Washington, D.C., James Slover, M.D., and his colleagues from Dartmouth Medical College reported on information gathered from more than 3,400 patients who had undergone back surgery. They found that factors such as depression, frequent headaches, and having a worker's compensation claim had a more powerful influence on patients' ability to function after back surgery than the presence of conditions such as heart disease or rheumatoid arthritis.

"There's the risk of focusing too much on the one particular anatomical problem when what influences quality of life is what's going on with the whole person," says Michael Von Korff, Sc.D., a researcher with Group Health Cooperative in Seattle who, with his colleagues, published an article about chronic back pain in the journal *PAIN* (February 2005). In it, they reported that nearly 90 percent of people with chronic back pain have at least one other chronic pain condition, chronic physical ailment, substance abuse problem, or mental disorder, such as diabetes, heart disease, rheumatoid arthritis, osteoporosis, depression, or cancer.

Although patients who do not have other health problems fare better after undergoing back surgery, even otherwise healthy individuals often do not get complete symptom relief or return to normal function, as you've already learned in this chapter. Thus, when it comes to making a decision about having back surgery, you and your physician should also consider the presence of other health problems you may have, as well as any emotional, social, and financial factors or motivators that could have a significant impact on the outcome of your surgery. Remember: *back surgery may not be a cure*. You will need to participate in rehabilitation, an exercise program, and/or other therapies not only as part of your healing process but likely for the rest of your life if you want to retain the benefits of your surgery.

You can greatly improve your chances of staying motivated to do these activities if you have a positive attitude and positive goals. For example,

- you want to return to activities you once enjoyed, such as dancing, hiking, volunteering at church, or playing with your grandchildren.
- you want to enjoy new activities that can be fun as well as therapeutic, such as tai chi, yoga, Jazzercise, Pilates, a walking club, or swimming.

- you plan to begin or return to traveling, whether that means day trips to the beach or plane or train travel to visit friends, family, or new places.
- if you have diabetes, hypertension, or heart disease, improved mobility after surgery will allow you to be more physically active, which may translate into better natural control of your health (e.g., stabilize blood sugar levels, lower blood pressure) and thus reduce your need for medications for these conditions.
- with increased mobility, less pain, and more energy, you will feel better able to advance your career, perhaps by taking classes or looking for a new job.
- once you have less pain, you'll sleep better, feel more self-confident, and want to take better care of yourself.

IN CONCLUSION . . .

If you are among the small minority of patients with chronic low back pain who need surgery, then you should take all the steps necessary to help ensure it is successful. I hope the information and guidelines I offered in this chapter help as you contemplate this important decision. Again, I urge you to seriously explore the treatment options I presented in previous chapters and solicit information from health-care professionals and other patients as part of your decision-making process.

Looking Ahead at Back Pain

There will always be a small percentage of cases of back pain that are not preventable: pain that is the result of accidental trauma; birth defects; or some other physical abnormality, infection, or disease. Some of the up-and-coming treatments and procedures that I talk about later in this chapter will likely be very helpful in these situations. But I believe that the future for you and others who have chronic low back pain can be a better, brighter, less painful one if you incorporate practices into your lifestyle that *we know work now*.

THE FUTURE IS NOW

First, let's review what you can do to treat chronic low back pain.

- Follow the recommendations in this book, especially the exercises, the movement therapies, and the body therapies.

- Learn the proper ways to lift (see the box below). If your work or other activities require you to lift heavy items, use a back support.
- Learn to sit and stand properly. Sitting places a great deal of pressure on the lower back, and sitting incorrectly can be a major contributor to back pain. Having the right chair (see chapter 4) can be critical, especially if you sit a great deal of the time. Movement therapies (e.g., Feldenkrais Method, Alexander Technique) and physical therapists can help you with posture and questions about sitting and standing.
- Regularly engage in activities that are both enjoyable and will help you improve posture and balance and/or enhance muscle strength and tone, such as tai chi, Pilates, walking, and yoga.
- Incorporate at least one stress-reduction practice into your life, such as meditation, yoga, visualization/guided imagery, progressive relaxation, or breathing therapy.
- If you are overweight, losing weight may take some of the stress off your lower back.
- Get seven to eight hours of sleep each night. Fatigued muscles are more prone to injury. If quality sleep is marred by a poor mattress, invest in a better one, if possible.

LIFTING GUIDELINES

- When lifting an object from the floor, stand close to the object and spread your feet to about shoulder width apart to give yourself a foundation of support. Bend your knees slightly, keep your back straight, and grasp the object. Hold the object close to your body as you straighten your legs and stand up.

- When you need to lift an object from a higher point, such as retrieving groceries from a car trunk or an infant from a crib, place one foot several inches behind the other. Lean forward and bend from your hips, lift the object, bring it close to you, and then stand up straight.

- An alternative way to lift objects from a point above the floor is to tighten your abdominal muscles, place one foot up on a footstool or other sturdy elevated object, and lean your forearms on the edge of the crib, table, cart, or trunk. As you lift up, bring the object close to your body and then straighten up.

- If you need to lift and twist (e.g., you are getting something from the bottom shelf in the refrigerator), squat and pull the item toward you. While you are in the squat position, twist and then stand up.

- Lift the object at a moderate speed using a smooth motion. If you lift an object too quickly, you can "jerk" the weight and/or lose control of the object. However, if you lift the object too slowly, you may lose balance as well. In either case, you risk muscle injury.

EMERGING THERAPIES

Several innovative therapies and techniques for treating back pain are either emerging or in the development stage. Here I will briefly discuss six of them: combination of robotics and minimally invasive surgery, artificial discs, making bone (osteoinduction), navigational imaging, disc nucleoplasty, and magnetic resonance neurography.

Minimally Invasive and Robotic Surgery

The use of minimally invasive surgery for back pain, such as laminectomy, discectomy, and spinal fusion, is gradually becoming commonplace as more surgeons are trained in this highly specialized surgical area. Laparoscopic surgery, the development of more advanced surgical cameras and other devices used in these procedures, and the introduction of robotics have the potential to dramatically change the outcome of back surgery. Robotic surgery, which as of this writing is not widely available, should enhance the accuracy of minimally invasive spine surgeries. Robotics will allow surgeons to make extremely precise and critical surgical moves without having to worry about hand tremors or fatigue. The combination of robotics and minimally invasive surgery should result in better results, less chance of infection and complications, faster recovery times, less hospitalization time, and most important, happier patients.

Artificial Discs

In October 2004, the first artificial discs were approved by the FDA for use in a new field of spine surgery called nonfusion or motion-preservation techniques. Unlike current spinal fusion surgery, in which vertebrae are fused together, thus preventing movement, the use of artificial discs will hopefully allow the spine to maintain movement. This means a spine that has artificial discs should function close to normal. The use of artificial discs, which are made of metal and/or polyethylene, will also reduce the risk of wear and tear on adjacent discs in the spine, which occurs with spinal fusion therapy (see Spinal Fusion in chapter 8), as well as eliminate the need for a bone graft and the risk of pain associated with pseudarthrosis (failure of a bone graft to fuse).

Although artificial discs are available, they are not yet widely used in the United States. Also, not everyone who is a candidate for spinal fusion is eligible for an artificial disc, at least not at this time. For now, eligible individuals must need only one disc replaced, and that disc must be between the fourth and fifth lumbar vertebrae or between the fifth lumbar vertebra and the sacrum. Candidates must have tried but failed at least six months of physical therapy, pain medication, or wearing a back brace, and they must be in otherwise good health (e.g., no arthritis, infection, or osteoporosis). Individuals who have significant leg pain also are not eligible.

Making Bone

As you may recall, spinal fusions require the transplantation of bone from the patient's pelvis to the vertebrae, a process that can prolong surgery, increase recovery time, result in increased pain during recovery, and increase blood loss. In an attempt to eliminate the need for bone transplantation, scientists have discovered that a genetically produced protein, recombinant human bone morphogenetic protein-2 (rhBMP-2), can stimulate the body's cells to make more bone. This process, called osteoinduction, can eliminate the need for bone transplantation from the pelvis and, as a bonus, may result in a faster, more reliable fusion.

The first clinical trial using rhBMP-2 was done in 1997 and included eleven patients. Ten of the patients achieved complete fusion within three months of surgery. At the end of 2001, physicians at the New Hampshire Spine Institute published an article about twenty-one patients (average age thirty-eight years) who underwent laparoscopic spinal fusion using rhBMP-2. At six and twelve months after the surgery, 100 percent of the patients reported relief of back pain, 100 percent had improved leg pain, and 100 percent said they had significant functional improvement. X-rays showed that all of the patients had a solid fusion at six months after surgery. So far, the use of both rhBMP-2 and laparoscopic surgery for spinal fusion has shown promising results, and the combination may soon be the preferred surgical approach.

Navigational Imaging

A technique called spinal navigational technology uses a combination of X-rays and computer assistance that allows surgeons to more accurately place surgical instruments, perform decompression, remove tumors, and do other surgical tasks. Rather than depend on CT or MRI scans that are done during preoperative testing, surgeons will be able to get real-time, three-dimensional images of a patient's spine on a computer screen right in the operating room, complete with virtual images of the surgical instruments the surgeons will be using. Surgeons will have the ability to plan the procedure, take measurements, and prepare for instrument placement, such as screws and rods, even before the patient is anesthetized. Overall, spinal navigation, along with minimally invasive techniques, will improve the outcome of back surgeries in the future.

Disc Nucleoplasty

This emerging procedure, which can be used to treat herniated discs that do not protrude beyond the outer wall, utilizes plasma energy (a method that uses low-temperature ionized particles) instead of heat energy to remove tissue from the center of a disc. Disc nucleoplasty is a minimally invasive surgery in which a needle is placed into the center of the affected disc and a wand is passed through the needle to the disc. The wand removes tissue from the disc and thus relieves the pressure. Thus far, the results of only a few studies have been reported, but the results are promising. In one study of eighty patients, 75 percent said they had reduced pain twelve months after undergoing the procedure. In another study, 82 percent of patients enjoyed greater than 50 percent pain reduction one year after the surgery.

The entire procedure takes about thirty minutes, and patients can go home shortly after surgery. Disc nucleoplasty may prove especially helpful for individuals with contained herniated discs who are unable to tolerate an open surgical procedure.

Magnetic Resonance Neurography

An emerging diagnostic tool is magnetic resonance (MR) neurography, which allows practitioners to see detailed images of nerves and locate those that may be damaged or irritated. This technology is important, as nerves cannot be seen on X-rays and are difficult to identify on CT scans, ultrasound, and regular MRI scans. The procedure for getting an MR neurogram is the same as it is for getting a regular MRI. The entire process takes thirty to forty minutes, and no contrast medium is required. However, the number of facilities that offer this test and the number of professionals who have been specially trained and who are proficient at it are still very limited.

IN CONCLUSION . . .

I applaud those people who have made the aforementioned strides in medical technology, and I believe the innovations discussed in this chapter will benefit many people who do or may someday experience chronic back pain. But as you know by now, I also am a strong advocate of natural, low-tech approaches to the treatment of back pain, especially when they have proven themselves again and again to be effective. I believe this will hold true tomorrow, just as it does today.

There's no time like the present to plan for your future. Strengthen and gently stretch your muscles. Learn how to stand, sit, sleep, lift, and move consciously and with the health of your back and your entire body in mind. Explore natural ways to manage stress and pain. Avoid or limit your use of medications. Have a positive attitude. And remember what your mother told you: sit up straight. Your back will thank you.

Notes

INTRODUCTION

Kostuik, John P., Suzanne M. Jan de Beur, and Simeon Margolis. *Johns Hopkins White Paper, Back Pain and Osteoporosis*, 2004.

Wheeler, A.H. et al. "Pathophysiology of Chronic Back Pain." At Emedicine, November 2004. http://www.emedicine.com/neuro/topic516.htm.

CHAPTER 1: YOUR ACHING BACK: WHY YOU HURT

Battie, M.C., T. Videman, E. Parent. "Lumbar Disc Degeneration: Epidemiology and Genetic Influences." *Spine* 2004 Dec 1; 29(23): 2679–90.

Brownstein, Art, M.D. *Healing Back Pain Naturally*. Gig Harbor, WA: Harbor Press, 1999.

Deyo, R.A., J.N. Weinstein. "Low Back Pain." *New England Journal of Medicine* 2001; 344: 363–70.

Dorland's Illustrated Medical Dictionary, 30th edition. Philadelphia: Saunders, 2001.

Froese, B.B. et al. "Lumbar Spondylolysis and Spondylolisthesis." At http://www.emedicine.com/pmr/topic69.htm.

Kapandji, I.A. *The Physiology of the Joints: The Trunk and Vertebral Column*, vol. 3. Edinburgh, UK: Churchill Livingstone, 1974.

Kenny, A., P. Taxel. "Osteoporosis in Older Men." *Clinical Cornerstone* 2000; 2: 45–51.

Lowe, Thomas G., M.D. "Degenerative Spondylolisthesis of the Lumbar Spine." At http://www.spineuniverse.com/displayarticle. php/article243.html.

Melton, L.J. 3d. "Epidemiology of Spinal Osteoporosis." *Spine* 1997; 22(24 Suppl): 2S–11S.

Melton, L.J. 3d et al. "Epidemiology of Vertebral Fractures in Women." *American Journal of Epidemiology* 1989; 129: 1000–11.

The Merck Manual of Health and Aging, "Compression Fractures of the Spine," at http://www.merck.com/pubs/mmanual_ha/ sec3/ch23/ch23c.html.

Mooney, V., J.A. Saal, J.S. Saal. "Evaluation and Treatment of Low Back Pain." *Clinical Symposia* 1996; 28 (4).

National Fibromyalgia Association, at http://www.fmaware.org/ fminfo/brochure.htm.

National Institute of Neurological Disorders and Stroke, National Institutes of Health. Back pain information Web page. At www.ninds.nih.gov/health_and_medical/disorders/backpain_doc. htm.

Resch, A. et al. "Risk of Vertebral Fractures in Men: Relationship to Mineral Density of the Vertebral Body." *American Journal of Roentgenology* 1995; 164: 1447–50.

Riggs, B.L., L.J. Melton. "The Worldwide Problem of Osteoporosis: Insights Afforded by Epidemiology." *Bone* 1995; 5: S505–S511.

Schwab, F. et al. "Adult Scoliosis: Prevalence SF-36, and Nutritional Parameters in an Elderly Volunteer Population." *Spine* 2005

1; 30(9): 1082–85. At http://www.spine-health.com/topics/cd/scoliosis/scoliosis01.html.

Sullivan, M.J., K. Reesor, S. Mikail, R. Fisher. "The Treatment of Depression in Chronic Low Back Pain: Review and Recommendations." *PAIN* 1992; 50: 5–13.

CHAPTER 2: GETTING HELP FOR YOUR CHRONIC BACK PAIN

American College of Rheumatology, criteria for fibromyalgia. At http://www.rheumatology.org/publications/classification/fibromyalgia/fibro.asp.

Cohen-Mansfield, J., M. Creedon. "Nursing Staff Members' Perceptions of Pain Indicators in Persons with Severe Dementia." *Clinical Journal of Pain* 2002; 18: 64–73.

Currie, S.R., J. Wang. "Chronic Back Pain and Major Depression in the General Canadian Population." *PAIN* 2004; 107: 54–60.

Deardorff, W.W. "Depression and Chronic Back Pain." At http://www.spinehealth.com/topics/cd/depression/depression01.html.

Jarvik, J.J., W. Hollingworth et al. "The Longitudinal Assessment of Imaging and Disability of the Back (LAIDBack) Study: Baseline Data." *Spine* 2001; 26(10): 1158–66.

Jensen, M.C. et al. "Magnetic Resonance Imaging of the Lumbar Spine in People Without Back Pain." *New England Journal of Medicine* 1994; 331: 69–73.

Kovach, C.R. et al. "The Assessment of Discomfort in Dementia Protocol." *Pain Management Nursing* 2002 Mar; 3(1): 16–27.

Kovach, C.R. et al. "Assessment and Treatment of Discomfort for People with Late-Stage Dementia." *Journal of Pain Symptom Management* 1999 Dec; 18(6): 412–19.

Patel, A.T., A.A. Ogle. "Diagnosis and Management of Acute Low Back Pain." *American Family Physician* 2000; 61(6): 1779–86, 1789–90. At www.aafp.org/afp/20000315/1779.html.

Perina, D. "Back Pain, Mechanical." At http://www.emedicine. com/EMERG/topic50.htm.

Sinel, M.S., W.W. Deardorff, T.B. Goldstein. In *Win the Battle Against Back Pain: An Integrated Mind-Body Approach*. New York: Bantam-Doubleday-Dell, 1996.

Sullivan, M.J. et al. "The Treatment of Depression in Chronic Low Back Pain: Review and Recommendations." *PAIN* 1992 July; 50(1): 5–13.

Waddell, G., D. Somerville, I. Henderson, M. Newton. "Objective Clinical Evaluation of Physical Impairment in Chronic Low Back Pain." *Spine* 1992; 17: 617–28.

Waddell, G. et al. "Nonorganic Physical Signs in Low-Back Pain." *Spine* 1980; 5: 117–25.

Wiesel, S.W. et al. "A Study of Computer-Assisted Tomography. I. The Incidence of Positive CAT Scans in an Asymptomatic Group of Patients." *Spine* 1994; 9: 549–51.

CHAPTER 3: STEP 1: LET'S GET PHYSICAL

Cacciatore, T.W., F.B. Horak, S.M. Henry. "Improvement in Automatic Postural Coordination Following Alexander Technique Lessons in a Person with Low Back Pain." *Physical Therapy* 2005 Jun; 85(6): 565–78.

Carroll, D., M. Tramer, H. McQuay. "Randomization Is Important in Studies with Pain Outcomes: Systematic Review of Transcutaneous Electrical Nerve Stimulation." *British Journal of Anesthesia* 1996; 77: 798–803.

Ernst, E., P.H. Canter. "The Alexander Technique: A Systematic Review of Controlled Clinical Trials." *Forsch Komplementarmed Klass Naturheilkd* 2003 Dec; 10(6): 325–29.

Fauno, P. et al. "Soreness in Lower Extremities and Back Is Reduced by Use of Shock Absorbing Heel Inserts." *International Journal of Sports Medicine* 1993; 14: 288–90.

Friberg, O. "Clinical Symptoms and Biomechanics of Lumbar Spine and Hip Joint in Leg Length Inequality." *Spine* 1983; 8: 643–51.

Giles, L.G.F., J.R. Taylor. "Low-Back Pain Associated with Leg Length Inequality." *Spine* 1981; 6: 510–21.

Giles, L.G.F., J.R. Taylor. "Lumbar Spine Structural Changes Associated with Leg Length Inequality." *Spine* 1982; 7: 159–62.

Hoffman, K.S., L.L. Hoffman. "Effects of Adding Sacral Base Leveling to Osteopathic Manipulative Treatment of Back Pain: A Pilot Study." *Journal of the American Osteopathic Association* 1994; 94: 217–26.

Hunter-Griffin, Letha Y. *Modalities: Athletic Training and Sports Medicine.* Park Ridge, IL: American Academy of Orthopaedic Surgeons, 1991.

Khadilkar, A. et al. "Transcutaneous Electrical Nerve Stimulation (TENS) for Chronic Low-Back Pain." *Cochrane Database of Systemic Reviews* 2005, Issue 3.

Light, L.H. et al. "Skeletal Transients on Heel Strike in Normal Walking with Different Footwear." *Journal of Biomechanics* 1980; 13: 477–80.

Yilmaz, F. et al. "Efficacy of Dynamic Lumbar Stabilization Exercise in Lumbar Microdiscectomy." *Journal of Rehabilitation Medicine* 2003 July; 35(4): 163–67.

CHAPTER 4: STEP 2: BODY THERAPIES

Ahmadi, S. et al. "Facilitation of Spinal NMDA Receptor Currents by Spillover of Synaptically Released Glycine." *Science* 2003 Jun 27; 300 (5628): 2094–97.

Andersson, G.B. et al. "A Comparison of Osteopathic Spinal Manipulation with Standard Care for Patients with Low Back Pain." *New England Journal of Medicine* 1999 Nov 4; 341(19): 1426–31.

The Better Sleep Council. "Bed Basics." 2003. At www.bettersleep.org/OnBetterSleep/bed_basics.asp; ConsumerReports.org.

"Mattress Sets." December 2002. At www.consumerreports.org/cro/home-garden/home-improvement/mattress-sets-buying-advice-206/index.htm.

Eisenberg et al. "Trends in Alternative Medicine Use in the United States, 1990–1997." *Journal of the American Medical Association* 1998 Nov 11; 280(18): 1569–75.

Galantino, M.L., T.M. Bzdewka et al. "The Impact of Modified Hatha Yoga on Chronic Low Back Pain: A Pilot Study." *Alternative Therapies in Health and Medicine* 2004 Mar-Apr; 10(2): 56–59.

Hass, C.J. et al. "The Influence of Tai Chi Training on the Center of Pressure Trajectory During Gait Initiation in Older Adults." *Archives of Physical Medicine and Rehabilitation* 2004 Oct; 85(10): 1593–98.

Hernandez-Reif, M., T. Field, J. Krasnegor, T. Theakston. "Low Back Pain Is Reduced and Range of Motion Increased After Massage Therapy." *International Journal of Neuroscience* 2001; 106: 131–45.

Kirkaldy-Willis, W.H., J.D. Cassidy. "Spinal Manipulation in the Treatment of Low Back Pain." *Canadian Family Physician* 1985; 31: 528–40.

Kovacs, F.M., V. Abraira et al. "Effect of Firmness of Mattress on Chronic Non-Specific Low-Back Pain: Randomized, Double-Blind, Controlled, Multicentre Trial." *Lancet* 2003 Nov 15; 362(9396): 1599–1604.

Li, F., P. Harmer, K.J. Fisher, E. McAuley. "Tai Chi: Improving Functional Balance and Predicting Subsequent Falls in Older Persons." *Medicine and Science in Sports and Exercise* 2004 Dec; 36(12): 2046–52.

Mandal, A.C. "Balanced Sitting Posture on Forward Sloping Seat." At www.acmandal.com.

"Public Attitudes Towards Massage Study," Caravan Opinion Research Corp., August 1999.

Qin, L. et al. "Beneficial Effects of Regular Tai Chi Exercise on

Musculoskeletal System." *Journal of Bone and Mineral Metabolism* 2005; 23(2): 186–90.

Thomas, K.J. et al. "Longer Term Clinical and Economic Benefits of Offering Acupuncture Care to Patients with Chronic Low Back Pain." *Health Technology Assessment* 2005 Aug; 9(32): 1–126.

Tsang, W.W., C.W. Hui-Chan. "Comparison of Muscle Torque, Balance, and Confidence in Older Tai Chi and Healthy Adults." *Medicine and Science in Sports and Exercise* 2005 Feb; 37(2): 280–89.

Tsang, W.W., C.W. Hui-Chan. "Effect of 4- and 8-week Intensive Tai Chi Training on Balance Control in the Elderly." *Medicine and Science in Sports and Exercise* 2004 Apr; 36(4): 648–57.

Wayne, P.M., D.E. Krebs et al. "Can Tai Chi Improve Vestibulopathic Postural Control?" *Archives of Physical Medicine and Rehabilitation* 2004 Jan; 85(1): 142–52.

Weiner, D. et al. "Efficacy of Percutaneous Electrical Nerve Stimulation for the Treatment of Chronic Low Back Pain in Older Adults." *Journal of American Geriatric Society* 2003 May; 51(5): 599–608.

Wiesinger, G.F. et al. "Benefit and Costs of Passive Modalities in Back Pain Outpatients: A Descriptive Study." *European Journal of Physical Medicine and Rehabilitation* 1997; 7: 182–86.

Williams, K.A., J. Petronis, D. Smith et al. "Effect of Iyengar Yoga Therapy for Chronic Low Back Pain." *PAIN* 2005 May; 115(1–2): 107–17.

Yeung, C.K., M.C. Leung, D.H. Chow. "The Use of Electroacupuncture in Conjunction with Exercise for the Treatment of Chronic Low-Back Pain." *Journal of Alternative and Complementary Medicine* 2003 Aug; 9(4): 479–90.

Yokoyama, M., X. Sun, S. Oku et al. "Comparison of Percutaneous Electrical Nerve Stimulation with Transcutaneous Electrical Nerve Stimulation for Long-Term Pain Relief in Patients with

Chronic Low Back Pain." *Anesthesia & Analgesia* 2004 Jun; 98(6): 1552–56.

CHAPTER 5: STEP 3: MINDING YOUR BACK

Baird, C.L., L. Sands. "A Pilot Study of the Effectiveness of Guided Imagery with Progressive Muscle Relaxation to Reduce Chronic Pain and Mobility Difficulties of Osteoarthritis." *PAIN Management Nursing* 2004 Sep; 5(3): 97–104.

Barnes, P.M. et al. "Complementary and Alternative Medicine Use Among Adults: United States, 2002." *Advance Data* 2004 May; 27 (343): 1–19.

Crawford, H.J. et al. "Hypnotic Analgesia: 1. Somatosensory Event-Related Potential Changes to Noxious Stimuli and 2. Transfer Learning to Reduce Chronic Low Back Pain." *International Journal of Clinical and Experimental Hypnosis* 1998 Jan; 46(1): 92–132.

Horton, J.E. et al. "Increased Anterior Corpus Callosum Size Associated Positively with Hypnotizability and the Ability to Control Pain." *Brain* 2004 Aug; 127(pt 8): 1741–47.

Kabat-Zinn, Jon, Ph.D. *Full Catastrophe Living*, chap. 5, at http://satipatthana.org/kabatzinn.html.

Lewandowski, W.A. "Patterning of Pain and Power with Guided Imagery." *Nursing Science Quarterly* 2004 Jul; 17(3): 233–41.

Mannix, L., D. Tusek, G. Solomon. "Effect of Guided Imagery on Quality of Life for Patients with Chronic Tension-Type Headache." *Headache: The Journal of Head and Face Pain* 1999 May; 39(5).

Mehling, W.E. "The Experience of Breath as a Therapeutic Intervention—Psychosomatic Forms of Breath Therapy. A Descriptive Study About the Actual Situation of Breath Therapy in Germany, Its Relation to Medicine, and Its Application in Patients with Back Pain." *Forsch Komplementarmed Klass Naturheilkd* 2001 Dec; 8(6): 359–67.

Mehling, W.E. et al. "Randomized, Controlled Trial of Breath Therapy for Patients with Chronic Low-Back Pain." *Alternative Therapies in Health and Medicine* 2005 Jul-Aug; 11(4): 44–52.

Newton-John, T.R., S.H. Spence, D. Schotte. "Cognitive-Behavioural Therapy Versus EMG Biofeedback in the Treatment of Chronic Low Back Pain." *Behaviour Research and Therapy* 1995 Jul; 33(6): 691–97.

NIH Technology Assessment Conference on the Integration of Behavioral and Relaxation Approaches into the Treatment of Chronic Pain and Insomnia. At http://www.hhs.gov/news/press/ 1995pres/951018b.html.

Ostelo, R.W. et al. "Behavioral Treatment for Chronic Low Back Pain." *Cochrane Database of Systematic Reviews* 2005 (1): CD002014.

Turner, J.A., S. Clancy. "Comparison of Operant-Behavioral and Cognitive-Behavioral Group Treatment for Chronic Low Back Pain." *Journal of Consulting and Clinical Psychology* 1988; 58: 573–79.

Van Tulder, M.W. et al. "Behavioral Treatment for Chronic Low Back Pain." *Cochrane Database of Systematic Reviews* 2000 (2): CD002014.

CHAPTER 6: STEP 4: GETTING THE POINT: INJECTION THERAPIES

Bryce, D.A., J. Nelson, I. Glurich, R.L. Berg. "Intradiscal Electrothermal Annuloplasty Therapy: A Case Series Study Leading to New Considerations." *Wisconsin Medical Journal* 2005 Aug; 104(6): 39–46.

Criscuolo, C.M. "Interventional Approaches to the Management of Myofascial Pain Syndrome." *Current Pain Headache Reports* 2001; 5: 407–11.

Davis, T.T. "The IDET Procedure for Chronic Discogenic Low Back Pain." *Spine* 2004; 29(7): 752–56.

Dreyfuss, P., M.D. "Lumbar Facet Joint Injections." At http://www.spineuniverse.com/displayarticle.php/article1176.html.

Dreyfuss, P., S.J. Dreyer, A. Cole, K. Mayo. "Sacroiliac Joint Pain." *Journal of the American Academy of Orthopaedic Surgeons* 2004; 12: 255–65.

Dreyfuss, P.H., S.J. Dreyer. "Lumbar Zygapophysial (Facet) Joint Injections." *The Spine Journal* 2003; 3(3Suppl): 50S–59S.

"Epidural Steroid Injections." At http://www.spine-health.com/topics/conserv/overview/inj/inj02.html.

Fine, P.G., R. Milano, B.D. Hare. "The Effects of Myofascial Trigger Point Injections Are Naloxone Reversible." *PAIN* 1988; 32(1): 15–20.

Garvey, T.A., M.R. Marks, S.W. Wiesel. "A Prospective, Randomized, Double-Blind Evaluation of Trigger Point Injection Therapy for Low Back Pain." *Spine* 1989; 14: 962–64.

Hauser, Ross, M.D. "What Is Prolotherapy?" At http://www.prolonews.com/what_is_prolotherapy.htm.

Hong, C.Z., T.C. Hsueh. "Difference in Pain Relief After Trigger Point Injections in Myofascial Pain Patients With and Without Fibromyalgia." *Archives of Physical Medicine and Rehabilitation* 1996; 77: 1161–66.

Hooper, R.A., M. Ding. "Retrospective Case Series on Patients with Chronic Spinal Pain Treated with Dextrose Prolotherapy." *Journal of Alternative and Complementary Medicine* 2004 Aug; 10(4): 670–74.

Klein, R.G., B.C. Eek, W.B. DeLong, V. Mooney. "A Randomized Double-Blind Trial of Dextrose-Glycerine-Phenol Injections for Chronic, Low Back Pain." *Journal of Spinal Disorders* 1993; 6: 23–33.

Lutz, C., G.E. Lutz, P.M. Cooke. "Treatment of Chronic Lumbar

Diskogenic Pain with Intradiscal Electrothermal Therapy: A Prospective Outcome Study." *Archives of Physical Medicine and Rehabilitation* 2003 Jan; 84(1): 23–28.

Melzack, R., P.D. Wall. "Pain Mechanisms: A New Theory." *Science* 1965; 150(699): 971–79.

Nash, T.P. "Facet Joints. Intraarticular Steroids or Nerve Blocks?" *Pain Clinic* 1990; 3: 77–82.

Ongley, M.J., R.G. Klein et al. "A New Approach to the Treatment of Chronic Low Back Pain." *Lancet* 1987; 2: 143–46.

Wagner, A.L. "Paraspinal Injection: Facet Joint and Nerve Root Blocks." At www.emedicine.com/radio/topic884.htm.

Yelland, M.J. et al. "Prolotherapy Injections, Saline Injections and Exercises for Chronic Low Back Pain: A Randomized Trial." *Spine* 2004 Jan 1; 29(1): 9–16.

Yelland, M.J. et al. "Prolotherapy Injections for Chronic Low Back Pain: A Systemic Review." *Spine* 2004 Oct 1; 29(19): 2126–33.

CHAPTER 7: STEP 5: MEET THE MEDS

Arkinstall, W., A. Sandler, B. Goughnour et al. "Efficacy of Controlled-Release Codeine in Chronic Non-Malignant Pain: A Randomized, Placebo-Controlled Clinical Trial." *PAIN* 1995; 62: 169–78.

Dellemijn, P.L., J.A. Vanneste. "Randomised Double-Blind Active-Placebo-Controlled Crossover Trial of Intravenous Fentanyl in Neuropathic Pain." *Lancet* 1997; 349: 753–58.

Moulin, D.E., A. Iezzi, R. Amireh et al. "Randomised Trial of Oral Morphine for Chronic Non-Cancer Pain." *Lancet* 1996; 347: 143–47.

National Institutes of Health press release. At http://www.nih .gov/news/pr/dec2004/od-17.htm.

National Library of Medicine. MedlinePlus article. "Drug Abuse and Dependence." At http://www.nlm.nih.gov/medlineplus/ency/article/001522.htm.

Nielsen, A.J. "Spray and Stretch for Myofascial Pain." *Physical Therapy* 1978; 58(5): 567–69.

Perina, D. "Back Pain, Mechanical." At http://www.emedicine.com/emerg/topic50.htm.

Ringe, J.D. et al. "Transdermal Fentanyl for the Treatment of Back Pain Caused by Vertebral Osteoporosis." *Rheumatology International* 2002 Sep; 22(5): 199–203.

Schug, S.A., A.F. Merry, R.H. Acland. "Treatment Principles for the Use of Opioids in Pain of Nonmalignant Origin." *Drugs* 1991; 42: 228–39.

Simpson, R.K., Jr., E.A. Edmondson, C.F. Constant et al. "Transdermal Fentanyl as Treatment for Chronic Low Back Pain." *Journal of Pain Symptom Management* 1997; 14: 218–24.

Turk, D.C., M.C. Brody, E.A. Okifuji. "Physicians' Attitudes and Practices Regarding the Long-Term Prescribing of Opioids for Non-Cancer Pain." *PAIN* 1994; 59: 201–8.

Van Tulder, M.W. et al. "Muscle Relaxants for Non-Specific Low-Back Pain." *Cochrane Database of Systematic Reviews* 2005, issue 3.

Watt, J.W., J.R. Wiles, D.R. Bowsher. "Epidural Morphine for Postherpetic Neuralgia." *Anesthesia* 1996; 51: 647–51.

CHAPTER 8: STEP 6: SURGERY AND OTHER INVASIVE TREATMENTS

Abitbol, J.J. "Vertebroplasty and Kyphoplasty: Treatment for Compression Fractures Resulting from Osteoporosis." At http://www.spineuniverse.com/displayarticle.php/article1525.html.

Auld, A.W., A. Maki-Jokela, D.M. Murdoch. "Intraspinal Narcotic Analgesia in the Treatment of Chronic Pain." *Spine* 1985; 10: 777–81.

Auld, A.W., D.M. Murdoch, K.A. O'Laughlin. "Intraspinal Narcotic Analgesia. Pain Management in Failed Laminectomy Syndrome." *Spine* 1987; 12: 953–54.

Barr, J.D., M.S. Barr, T.J. Lemley, R.M. McCann. "Percutaneous Vertebroplasty for Pain Relief and Spinal Stabilization." *Spine* 2000; 25: 923–28.

De la Porte, C., E. Van de Kelft. "Spinal Cord Stimulation in Failed Back Surgery Syndrome." *PAIN* 1993; 52(1): 55–61.

"The Evolving Role of the Surgeon in Back Pain Management: The New Care Continuum," a Medscape CME. At www.medscape.com/viewprogram/3171_pnt.

Grados, F., C. Depriester, G. Cayrolle et al. "Long-Term Observations of Vertebral Osteoporotic Fractures Treated by Percutaneous Vertebroplasty." *Rheumatology* 2000; 39: 1410–14.

Graz, B. et al. "Prognosis or 'Curabo Effect'? Physician Prediction and Patient Outcome of Surgery for Low Back Pain and Sciatica." *Spine* 2005 Jun 15; 30(12): 1448–52.

Jensen, M.E., A.J. Evans, J.M. Mathis et al. "Percutaneous Polymethylmethacrylate Vertebroplasty in the Treatment of Osteoporotic Vertebral Body Compression Fractures: Technical Aspects." *American Journal of Neuroradiology* 1997; 18: 1897–1904.

Krames, E.S., R.M. Lansing. "Intrathecal Infusional Analgesia for Nonmalignant Pain: Analgesic Efficacy of Intrathecal Opioid With or Without Bupivacaine." *Journal of Pain Symptom Management* 1993; 8: 539–48.

Lieberman, I.H. et al. "Initial Outcome and Efficacy of Kyphoplasty in the Treatment of Painful Osteoporotic Vertebral Compression Fractures." *Spine* Jul 2001; 26(14): 1631–38.

Lieberman, I.H., M.D. "Kyphoplasty: A New Treatment for Osteoporotic Vertebral Compression Fractures." At http://www.spine-universe.com/displayarticle.php/article181.html.

McGraw, J.K. et al. "Prospective Evaluation of Pain Relief in 100

Patients Undergoing Percutaneous Vertebroplasty: Results and Follow-up." *Journal of Vascular and Intervenioral Radiology* 2002; 13: 883–86.

Mehbod, A., S. Aunoble, J.C. LeHuec. "Vertebroplasty for Osteoporotic Spine Fracture: Prevention and Treatment." *European Spine Journal* 2003; 12 (Suppl 2): S155–S162.

Mooney, V., J.F. Saal, J.S. Saal. "Evaluation and Treatment of Low Back Pain." *Clinical Symposia* vol. 48 (4): 1996, p. 25.

Nelson, Colin. "Surgery Often Won't Cure Back Pain." WebMD article, Feb. 25, 2005. At http://my.webmd.com/content/Article/101/106112.htm?pagenumber=2.

"Nonsmokers Fare Better Than Smokers in Fusion Procedures," *Orthopedics Today* 2000 May; 20(5): 12.

North, R.B., M.G. Ewend, M.T. Lawton et al. "Failed Back Surgery Syndrome: 5-Year Follow-up After Spinal Cord Stimulator Implantation." *Neurosurgery* 1991; 28(5): 692–99.

North American Spine Society. "Open Discectomy." At http://www.spine.org/articles/discectomy.cfm.

North American Spine Society. "Spinal Fusion Surgery." At http://www.spine.org/articles/spinalfusion.cfm.

Peh, W., L. Gilula, D. Peck. "Percutaneous Vertebroplasty for Severe Osteoporotic Vertebral Body Compression Fractures." *Radiology* 2002; 223: 121–26.

Perez-Higueras, A., L. Alvarez, R.E. Rossi et al. "Percutaneous Vertebroplasty: Long Term Clinical and Radiological Outcome." *Neuroradiology* 2002; 44: 950–54.

Turner, J.A., J.D. Loeser, K.G. Bell. "Spinal Cord Stimulation for Chronic Low Back Pain: A Systematic Literature Synthesis." *Neurosurgery* 1995; 37(6): 1088–96.

Ullrich, Peter F., M.D. "Failed Back Surgery Syndrome." At http://www.spine-health.com/topics/surg/failed_back/failed_back05.html.

Von Korff, M. et al. "Chronic Spinal Pain and Physical-Mental Comorbidity in the United States: Results from the National Comorbidity Survey Replication." *PAIN* 2005 Feb; 113(3): 331–39.

Yoem, J.S. et al. "Percutaneous Transpedicular Vertebroplasty: Two-Year Follow-up Results of 38 Cases." Presented as poster exhibit at the Annual Meeting of the American Academy of Orthopaedic Surgeons. 2003 Feb 5–9; New Orleans.

EPILOGUE: LOOKING AHEAD AT BACK PAIN

American Association of Neurological Surgeons. "Artificial Disc Surgery an Option for Select Patients." At http://www.newswise.com/articles/view/513567/?sc=mwtn.

Kleeman, T.J., U.M. Ahn, A. Talbot-Kleeman. "Laparoscopic Anterior Lumbar Interbody Fusion with rhBMP-2: A Prospective Study of Clinical and Radiographic Outcomes." *Spine* 2001; 26: 2751–56.

Sandhu, H.S., M.D. "The Latest in Bone Growth Enhancement for Spinal Fusion." At http://www.spineuniverse.com/displayarticle.php/article1544.html.

Sharps, L., Z. Isaac. "Percutaneous Disc Decompression Using Nucleoplasty." *Pain Physician* 2002; 5(2): 121–26.

Singh, V., C. Piryani, K. Liao. "Evaluation of Percutaneous Disc Decompression Using Coblation in Chronic Back Pain With or Without Leg Pain." *Pain Physician* 2003; 6: 273–80.

Glossary

Acupoints: Acupuncture points located along channels on the surface of the body called meridians.

Acupuncture: A treatment approach in which a practitioner balances the vital energy in the body by inserting fine needles into specific acupoints, which in turn relieves pain and tension.

Addiction: A pattern of compulsive drug use characterized by a continued craving for a drug and the need to use the drug for effects other than pain relief.

Alexander Technique: A form of movement therapy in which teachers instruct individuals on proper posture, coordination, and muscle balance.

Analgesic: A medication that is used to relieve pain without causing a loss of consciousness, such as ibuprofen or aspirin.

Ankylosing spondylitis: A chronic, progressive arthritic disease of the joints that mainly affects the back, specifically the sacroiliac area, hip joints, and lumbar spine. *Ankylosing* refers to stiffness and immobility of a joint, while *spondylitis* refers to inflammation of one or more vertebrae.

Annulus: The outer covering of a disc.

Back extension: A backward bending of the spine.

Back flexion: A forward bending of the spine.

Biofeedback: Technique in which individuals practice different relaxation methods while using electronic sensing devices that measure their body functions, which allows them to hear or see how their body responds physically to stress. They can then learn how to consciously cause beneficial physical changes.

Breathing therapy: A general term for various breathing techniques individuals can use to relieve pain, tension, and stress.

Bulging disc: Abnormal protrusion of a vertebral disc from its normal position in the vertebral column in the setting of an intact but weakened annulus that may or may not be associated with pain.

Cartilage: A type of stiff yet flexible body tissue that forms the discs in the spine and many other joints throughout the body.

Cauda equina: The bundle of nerve roots located at the bottom of the spinal cord.

Chiropractic: A science based on the theory that health and disease are intimately associated with the nervous system and that an aligned spine is essential for health. Chiropractic involves the use of spinal manipulation, the application of heat or cold, massage, and electrical stimulation to treat back and other physical problems.

Chronic pain: Pain that lasts for more than three months. Generally, it limits an individual's ability to function fully and has both psychological and emotional effects.

Compressed nerve: A condition in which a nerve is pressed against the spinal cord by the material from a bulging or herniated disc or in which the nerve is pinched by arthritis as it exits the spinal column. This condition may be very painful or associated with no symptoms.

Compression fracture: Fracture of a vertebra that results in the loss of height or the complete collapse of the vertebral body. This type of fracture is usually associated with osteoporosis.

Computed tomography (CT): Imaging technique in which X-rays are passed through the body and sensed by a detector that rotates completely around the patient. A computer then compiles the information and creates a cross-sectional image that shows body structures and fluids.

Degenerative disc disease: A general term for a condition in which there is a deterioration of one or more spinal discs that may or may not cause symptoms.

Discectomy: A surgical procedure for treatment of a herniated disc in which part or all of a disc is removed to take pressure off a pinched nerve.

Dura mater: A tough fibrous membrane that covers the spinal cord and brain and is separated from them by a small space.

Epidural: Referring to the area located within the spinal canal, on or outside the dura mater.

Extensor muscles: Four muscles that originate on the vertebrae and extend vertically along the spine. Their purpose is to stabilize and extend the spine.

Facet joints: Joints at the back of each vertebra that link the vertebrae together.

Facet joint syndrome: A painful condition associated with degeneration of the facet joints.

Fascia: Connective tissue that separates muscles and organs in the body.

Fibromyalgia: A condition that is characterized by generalized pain that patients experience in muscles, ligaments, tendons, and joints and is associated with the nervous system processing pain abnormally.

Herniated disc: Condition in which the nucleus of a lumbar disc protrudes through the outer disc wall into the spinal canal and presses against a nerve, which can result in severe pain.

Infusion: A method of giving pain medication into a vein or under the skin. Unlike an injection, which is given by a syringe, an infusion flows by gravity or is given using a mechanical pump.

Intervertebral disc: The flexible pad of tissue located between the vertebrae that acts as a shock absorber or cushion and prevents the vertebrae from grinding against each other. Also referred to simply as a disc.

Kyphoplasty: Surgical technique to treat vertebral compression fractures in which the collapsed vertebra is expanded using a special balloon and then filled with cement.

Kyphosis: Condition in which the upper back is severely rounded. Also known as a hunchback.

Lamina: The posterior part of the vertebral arch.

Laminectomy: Surgical procedure in which the lamina is removed for the purpose of relieving pain caused by compression of a nerve from a slipped or herniated disc or to treat spinal stenosis.

Ligament: A band of fibrous tissue that connects bones or cartilage and supports the joints.

Lordosis: An abnormal, concave curve of the spine. Also known as swayback.

Lumbar spine: Area of the back also referred to as the lower back; it is composed of five weight-bearing vertebrae located between the thoracic vertebrae and the sacrum.

Magnetic resonance imaging (MRI): A highly sensitive imaging technique in which a powerful magnet surrounds the patient while radio waves are passed through the body. No X-rays are involved.

Massage therapy: A general term used to describe various bodywork techniques, such as Swedish massage and shiatsu.

Meditation: A general term used to describe numerous practices in which you focus your awareness on one thing, such as breath, an object, or a sound, in order to quiet the mind.

Microdiscectomy: A surgical treatment for herniated discs that is less invasive than a discectomy because it is performed through a smaller incision.

Muscle spasm: A sudden, often severe, involuntary contraction of a muscle or group of muscles that is accompanied by pain and disrupted function.

Myofascial pain: A common, painful disorder that can affect any of the skeletal muscles in the body and is characterized by the presence of trigger points, which are hypersensitive spots within muscles. It can cause local or referred pain, tenderness, limited mobility, tightness, popping and clicking, and weakness.

Myofascial release: Use of gentle stretching and massage to ease pressure in the fascia (the sheath that covers muscle).

Nerve block: A pain-relief method in which an anesthetic is injected into a nerve.

Nerve root: The part of the nerve that exits the spinal canal and extends beyond the vertebrae.

Neurosurgeon: A physician who specializes in surgery on the brain, spinal cord, and nerves.

Neurotransmitters: Substances that are released by nerves to transmit signals to other nerves or to the brain.

Nonprescription (over-the-counter): Medications that can be obtained without a doctor's prescription.

Nucleus: The inner core of a disc.

Opioid: Any of various painkilling drugs that contain opium or one or more of its natural or synthetic derivatives. Opioids are also called narcotics.

Osteoporosis: A disease characterized by loss of bone density, resulting in brittle and/or porous bones and commonly affecting the vertebrae and hip bones.

Palpation: Use of the hands during a physical examination to feel for abnormalities.

Percutaneous electrical nerve stimulation (PENS): Treatment technique that combines acupuncture needles with varying levels of electrical stimulation. It is based on the structure of the nervous system, not on meridians (acupuncture channels).

Physiatrist: A medical doctor who specializes in problems of the bones and muscles and focuses on rehabilitation rather than on surgery.

Physical therapy: Health profession that treats pain with exercise, hydrotherapy, bodywork (e.g., massage), electrical stimulation, heat, cold, and other methods.

Piriformis muscle: A muscle that begins at the sacrum and attaches to the top outer part of the thigh bone. *See* piriformis syndrome.

Piriformis syndrome: Condition that occurs when the piriformis muscle compresses the sciatic nerve and irritates it, causing sciatica. The pain of piriformis syndrome increases with the contraction of the piriformis muscle, prolonged sitting, or direct pressure on the muscle.

Prolapsed disc: Another name for a herniated disc.

Radiculopathy: Pain that radiates away from the originating point in the spine. A common cause of radiculopathy is deformity of one or more discs that presses on a spinal nerve.

Rhizotomy: Incision of nerve roots in the spinal cord.

Ruptured disc: Another name for a herniated disc.

Sacroiliac (SI) joint: The joint located between the sacrum and pelvis; there are two SI joints, one on each side.

Sacroiliac joint syndrome: Pain produced by a strain of the sacroiliac joint.

Sacrum: The flat, triangular bone located at the base of the spine.

Sciatica: A condition characterized by pain along the course of the sciatic nerve, which runs from the back down through the buttocks and into the leg. The pain may be accompanied by numbness and/or tingling.

Scoliosis: Abnormal curving of the spine to the side, which is apparent when viewed from behind.

Slipped disc: Another name for a herniated disc.

Spinal canal: Channel through which the spinal cord runs. It is formed by the bony arch of each vertebra.

Spinal fusion: A surgical procedure in which bone grafts are used to attach two or more adjacent vertebrae to each other.

Spinal stenosis: A narrowing of the spinal canal, which causes pressure to build against a nerve or against the spinal cord.

Spondylitis: Inflammation of the vertebrae, sometimes caused by an infection.

Spondylolisthesis: Condition in which an individual vertebra slips forward or backward over the one below it.

Spondylosis: Condition characterized by degeneration of the vertebrae, discs, and facet joints.

Sprain: Overstretch or tearing injury of a ligament.

Strain: Overstretching, twisting, or pulling of a muscle or tendon.

Tai chi: A meditative movement form that emphasizes gentle, slow, flowing motion. It is helpful in building and maintaining balance and good posture and in reducing stress.

Tensor fascia lata: A muscle on the side of the hip that starts from the top of the iliac crest and ends on the iliotibial band (band of connective tissue on the side of the thigh); it flexes the hip and helps to stabilize the leg when a person is standing.

Tolerance: Decreasing effect of a drug when it is taken at the same dose, or the need to increase the dose of the drug to maintain the same effect.

Transcutaneous electrical nerve stimulation (TENS): Treatment technique in which low-energy electrical signals are transmitted to interrupt the transmission of pain signals in the nerves.

Trigger point: A hyperirritable area in a muscle that arises with myofascial pain.

Trigger point therapy: Technique in which pressure is applied to specific trigger points in the muscles to relieve pain and tension.

Ultrasound: Treatment technique in which high-frequency sound waves are used to generate heat below the surface of the skin. It is also a diagnostic tool used to detect osteoporosis and fractures.

Vertebrae: The series of thirty-three bones that make up the spinal column.

Vertebroplasty: Surgical technique to treat vertebral compression fractures in which the collapsed vertebra is injected with cement.

Resources

―――― ❦ ――――

THERAPEUTIC APPROACHES

Acupuncture
American Academy of Medical Acupuncture
4929 Wilshire Blvd, Ste 428
Los Angeles CA 90010
323-937-5514
www.medicalacupuncture.org

Alexander Technique
Alexander Technique International
U.S. Office: 1692 Massachusetts Ave, 3rd floor
Cambridge MA 02138
1-888-668-8996

Biofeedback
Association for Applied Psychophysiology and Biofeedback
10200 W 44th Ave, Ste 304
Wheat Ridge CO 80033
1-800-477-8892
www.aapb.org

Breath Therapy

Heart Centered Therapies Association
3716 274th Ave SE
Issaquah WA 98029
1-800-914-8348
www.heartcenteredtherapies.org

Chiropractic

American Chiropractic Association
1701 Clarendon Blvd
Arlington VA 22209
1-800-986-4636
www.amerchiro.org

Cognitive-Behavior Therapy

National Association of Cognitive-Behavioral Therapists
PO Box 2195
Weirton WV 26062
1-800-853-1135
www.nacbt.org

Feldenkrais Method

Feldenkrais Educational Foundation of North America
3611 SW Hood Ave, Ste 100
Portland OR 97239
1-866-333-6248
www.feldenkrais.com

Heart Centered Therapies Association

3716 274th Ave SE
Issaquah WA 98029
1-800-914-8348
www.heartcenteredtherapies.org

Massage

American Massage Therapy Association
500 David St, Ste 900
Evanston IL 60201
1-877-905-2700
www.amtamassage.org

McKenzie Method

McKenzie Institute
126 N Salina St
Syracuse NY 13202
315-471-7612
www.mckenziemdt.org/index_us.cfm

Meditation

Center for Mindfulness in Medicine, Health Care, and Society
55 Lake Avenue North
Worcester MA 01655
508-856-2656
www.umassmed.edu

Meditation Society of America
PO Box 126
Wagontown PA 19376
www.meditationsociety.com

Pilates

Pilates Method Alliance
PO Box 370906
Miami FL 33137-0906
1-866-573-4945
www.pilatesmethodalliance.org

Self-Hypnosis
American Society of Clinical Hypnosis
140 N Bloomingdale Rd
Bloomingdale IL 60108
630-980-4740
www.asch.net

Visualization/Guided Imagery
Academy for Guided Imagery
PO Box 2070
Mill Valley CA 94942
415-389-9324
www.academyforguidedimagery.com

Yoga
American Yoga Association
PO Box 19986
Sarasota FL 34276
941-927-4977
www.americanyogaassociation.org

GENERAL

American Academy of Pain Medicine
4700 W Lake
Glenview IL 60025
847-375-4731
www.painmed.org

American Association of Neurological Surgeons
5550 Meadowbrook Dr
Rolling Meadows IL 60008
1-888-566-2267
www.aans.org

American Chronic Pain Association
PO Box 850
Rocklin CA 95677-0850
1-800-533-3231
www.theacpa.org

American Pain Foundation
201 N Charles St, Ste 710
Baltimore MD 21201
1-888-615-7246
www.painfoundation.org

American Pain Society
4700 West Lake Ave
Glenview IL 60025
847-375-4715
www.ampainsoc.org

International Association for the Study of Pain
111 Queen Anne Avenue N, Ste 501
Seattle WA 98109
206-283-3011
www.iasp-pain.org

National Chronic Pain Outreach Association
PO Box 274
Millboro VA 24460
540-862-9437
www.chronicpain.org

National Institute of Health
Osteoporosis and Related Bone Disease National Resource
Center
2 AMS Circle
Bethesda MD 20892
1-800-624-BONE
www.osteo.org

National Osteoporosis Foundation
1232 22nd St NW
Washington DC 20037
202-223-2226

National Pain Foundation
300 E Hampden Ave, Ste 100
Englewood CO 80113
E-mail: aardrup@nationalpainfoundation.org
www.painconnection.org

Pain Management Clinics
www.pain.com
Provides a list of pain management clinics by state

FOR INTEGRATIVE PRACTITIONER REFERRALS

**Health World, Directory to Find Integrative Health
Professionals**
www.healthy.net/scr/center.asp?centerid=53

Suggested Reading and Videos/DVDs

Achterberg, Jeanne. *Rituals of Health: Using Imagery for Health and Wellness.* New York: Bantam, 1994.

Alman, Brian, and Peter Lambrou. *Self-Hypnosis: The Complete Manual for Health and Self-Change.* New York: Brunner-Routledge, 1992.

Angell, Marcia. *The Truth About Drug Companies: How They Deceive Us and What to Do About It.* New York: Random House, 2004.

Arthritis Foundation of America. *All You Need to Know About Back Pain.* Atlanta, GA: Arthritis Foundation of America, 2002.

Benson, Herbert. *The Relaxation Response.* New York: Avon Books, 1975.

Borysenko, Joan. *Minding the Body, Mending the Mind.* New York: Bantam, 1987.

Brownstein, Art, M.D. *Healing Back Pain Naturally.* Gig Harbor, WA: Harbor Press, 1999.

Christensen, Alice. *American Yoga Association Beginner's Manual.* New York: Fireside, 1987.

Christensen, Alice. *The American Yoga Association's Easy Does It Yoga.* New York: Fireside, 1999.

Dossey, Larry, M.D. *Healing Words.* San Francisco: Harper, 1993.

Fishman, Loren M., and Carol Ardman. *Relief Is in the Stretch: End Back Pain Through Yoga.* New York: WW Norton, 2005.

Gawain, Shakti. *The Complete Creative Visualization Workbook.* Novato, CA: New World Library, 1995.

Gawain, Shakti. *Creative Visualization.* 25th anniversary ed. Novato, CA: New World Library, 2002.

Kabat-Zinn, Jon. *Full Catastrophe Living: Using the Wisdom of Your Body and Mind to Face Stress, Pain, and Illness.* New York: Doubleday/Dell, 1990.

Kidson, Ruth. *Acupuncture for Everyone: What It Is, Why It Works and How It Can Help You.* Rochester, VT: Healing Arts Press, 2001.

Lam, Paul. *Tai Chi for Back Pain: Also for Wheelchair Bound and Other Chronic Conditions.* Narwee, NSW: Tai Chi Productions, 2004 (DVD).

Levin-Gervasi, Stephanie. *The Back Pain Sourcebook.* New York: McGraw-Hill, 1998.

Lidell, Lucinda. *Book of Massage: Complete Step-by-Step Guide.* New York: Simon & Schuster, 1984, 2001.

McKenzie, Eleanor. *The Joseph H. Pilates Method at Home.* Berkeley, CA: Ulysses Press, 2000.

McKenzie, Robin. *7 Steps to a Pain-Free Life: How to Rapidly Relieve Back and Neck Pain Using the McKenzie Method.* New York: Plume Books, 2001.

Medical Economics Inc. *The PDR Family Guide to Prescription Drugs.* 9th ed. Three Rivers Press, 2002.

Miller, Fred L. *How to Calm Down: Three Deep Breaths to Peace of Mind.* New York: Warner, 2003.

Miller, Fred L. *Yoga: For Common Aches and Pains.* New York: Perigee, 2004.

Miller, Robert. *Back Pain Relief: The Ultimate Guide.* Santa Barbara: Capra Press, 1997.

Monro, Robin, R. Nagarantha, and H.R. Nagendra. *Yoga for Common Ailments.* New York: Fireside Books, 1990.

Naparstek, Belleruth. *Staying Well with Guided Imagery.* New York: Warner, 1995.

Pilates, Joseph. *The Pilates' Primer: The Millennium Edition.* Talent, OR: Presentation Dynamics, 2000.

Rossman, Martin L., M.D. *Guided Imagery for Self-Healing.* Novato, CA: New World Library, 2000.

Rybacki, James J. *The Essential Guide to Prescription Drugs 2005.* New York: Collins, 2004.

Sarno, John, M.D. *Healing Back Pain.* New York: Warner Books, 1991.

Schatz, Mary Pullig, M.D. *Back Care Basics: A Doctor's Gentle Yoga Program for Back and Neck Pain Relief.* Berkeley, CA: Rodmell Press, 1992.

Sobel, Dava, and Arthur C. Klein. *Backache: What Exercises Work.* New York: St. Martin's, 1994.

Sollars, David W. *Complete Idiot's Guide to Acupuncture and Acupressure.* New York: Alpha, 2000.

Stanmore, Tia. *Spine Work: Pilates Based Exercises for Neck, Back and Shoulders.* London: Hamlyn, 2002.

Swayzee, Nancy. *Breathworks for Your Back.* New York: Avon Books, 1998.

Thomas, Sara. *Massage for Common Ailments.* New York: Simon & Schuster, 1989.

Weil, Andrew, and Martin L. Rossman. *Self-Healing with Guided Imagery: How to Use the Power of Your Mind to Heal Your Body.* Audio CD. Sounds True, 2004.

Weller, Stella. *The Yoga Back Book: The Gentle Yet Effective Way to Spinal Health.* London: Thorsons, 2000.

Wolfe, Sidney M. *Worst Pills, Best Pills: A Consumer's Guide to Avoiding Drug-Induced Death or Illness.* New York: Pocket, 2005.

Index